Sick and Tired & sexy

Living Beautifully with Chronic Illness

Donna O'Klock

TREATY OAK PUBLISHERS

Dedication

For Turk -
Without you, I would have only dreamt.

In Memory

Evelyn, Terry, Russ, Teresa, Nancy, and Josh

Publisher's Note

Printed and published in the United States of America

Treaty Oak Publishers

ISBN-13: 978-1-943658-11-4
ISBN-10: 1-943658-11-0

Sick and Tired & Sexy

Living Beautifully with Chronic Illness

I set out to make a difference to people who are on the same path as me."

- Seth Godin

Chronically pushing away your experience will lead to chronically feeling tired."

- Tara Mohr

Table of Contents

Part Two - Staying There

Section 1

Section 2

INTRODUCTION

Introduction

First, let's talk about "sexy" for a second, since it is a major component of this book. While it's challenging enough to maintain a great relationship with yourself, and with a partner, when you are well, it's exponentially more challenging when you're feeling sick and tired all of the time. And, almost without exception, the sexy side of ourselves seems to be the first thing we let fall by the wayside when we become ill. Believe me, I understand. Who has energy or desire when they are sick?

But, in order to feel well, it's the sexy part of our being that we will need to tap into and treat with the respect and care it deserves. Knowing what you want, and what you are going to do to make it happen, is sexy. Sexy as in confident, self-possessed, and comfortable-in-our-skin. Sexy as in giving-a-damn, saying to yourself, "I've got this!" Caring about how you show up in your world is sexy.

Although I'm no youngster, that sexy side of myself was not something I was ready or willing to give up, even though I hadn't seen hide-nor-hair of it in months. I made a conscious decision to care about looking better than the zombie I felt like. Looking better made me feel better, which gave me a tad more energy. I felt more able, and that made me feel even better, creating an upward spiral.

While my relationship benefited from this improvement, I'm definitely the one who benefited most, especially when I walked past a mirror. After months of feeling horrid and avoiding mirrors, I remember seeing myself one day and thinking, "Hmmnnn... I don't look nearly as bad as I feel!

> " *Whatever you can do, or dream you can, begin it. Boldness has genius, power, and magic in it.*"
>
> - Johann Goethe

Realizing I could change my life for the better led me to taking my first step: I made a plan to begin each day inspired. Actually, that was my second step, right after taking a shower and throwing my hoodie and sweat pants into the trash. I spent 30-60 minutes each morning reading, watching videos, or listening to something inspiring, informative, or educational.

I sought out people with different things to offer me: Tony Robbins. Danielle LaPorte. Marie Forleo. Ina Garten. Linda Sivertsen. Seth Godin. Marianne Williamson. Louise Hay. The Dalai Lama. Julia Cameron. Dr. Wayne Dyer. Sir Richard Branson. Liz Gilbert. Deepak Choprah. Mark Sisson. Ann Lamott. Dr. Andrew Weil. The Gluten-Free Goddess. Oprah Winfrey. Ellen DeGeneres. And the TED Talks.

I also followed, with a touch of envy, the trajectory of a dear friend as he succeeded in fulfilling his dream. Following Ted's success as a "stylist to the stars" reminded me that I used to have a dream also, and it had been left on the shelf for far too long. My joy for his creative success pointed me toward my own dream. I've since wondered if getting that sick was what it took for me to follow my heartfelt desire.

I began making my bed first thing every morning. By doing this, I signaled to my subconscious that I was ready to begin my day. There was also the added benefit of how polished the bedroom looked for the first time in a long time. In the grander scheme, it signaled my belief that I was well enough to get out of bed and get on with living my life.

For the first month of my plan, I still spent most of the day on the couch, but I was showered, dressed, and seeking inspiration. I had quit resenting the circumstances

I found myself in, and chose instead to make the best of them. After a week or so, rather than feeling depressed, I now felt hopeful.

I resumed a daily writing practice that began by creating a wellness journal to keep track of what was working, and what wasn't. I slowly took a more active part in my medical care by asking lots more questions, doing research, trying different things, and keeping good records. I was beginning to feel like an equal-partner, rather than just a patient.

All of these internal changes eventually manifested themselves externally. I changed how and what I was eating. I changed how I dressed, I simplified my makeup, and decided on a chic hairstyle that suited my new "medically induced" hair. Over time, all of this became ingrained, and turned into My Life, version 2.0.

" *If you're going through hell, keep going!"*

- Winston Churchill

Last month, I met my new primary care doctor. She walked in the room, stopped, and looked me in the eye. "Wow! I checked your age, your medical history, and the list of meds on your chart… and I had a completely different mental picture of what you would look like. You look great!"

I was flattered, not because I'm vain, (well, maybe a little bit) but because it means the choices I make every day are working.

For 35 years I worked in the beauty industry, and my goal was always to make people look and feel beautiful. I kept them up on current trends and shared what I knew on a wide variety of topics that related to wellness and beauty. When I became seriously ill, I had to sit in my own chair and use those same skills to help myself build a new life, one that included chronic illnesses.

In spite of the current trend toward life-hacks, and a how-to-do-almost-anything-in-seven-easy-steps, I have to tell you upfront, there are no shortcuts. There is only doing your work.

In these pages I share what worked for me, backed by my lifelong pursuit of personal growth, my belief in the connection of our body, mind, and spirit, and in a responsive Universe. I share my experiences with alternative wellness practitioners who are becoming mainstream now. And I talk about my life-long commitment to nutritious food, and the necessity (and joy) of physical activity.

You'll notice ideas will be repeated and will overlap. Everything in the book is interwoven and works synergistically with everything else. And just like life, where opportunity doesn't only knock once, themes will recur in different chapters allowing ideas that may not have resonated for you the first time to be viewed in another context. The light bulb can be turned on and you will see how you can apply it to your life.

Everything is meant to give you the energy and inspiration you need to feel sexy and live beautifully again. If you're still lying on the couch wondering how the hell to get up and get your life back, my hope is that **Sick and Tired** … & *Sexy* will get you started on your way.

With love and respect for your journey,

XO Donna

PREFACE

Preface

I had everything I ever wanted: work I enjoyed, a darling fiancé, a house with a pool, and exciting motorcycle trips around the country with friends. Our children were now grown and on their own. So, what was the problem?

I couldn't get up off of the couch to enjoy any of it.

I'd lost track of how many weeks I'd been lying on that couch. My sweetheart had been so patient, always considerate and concerned. One day he walked into the living room and said, "Honey, why don't you get up and take a shower?"

Smiling down at me, hopeful, he added, "You'll feel so much better."

"I really can't. You don't understand, I'm so exhausted, I'd probably drown. Like a turkey in a rainstorm."

"Well, okay, if you don't have any more sense than that." Chuckling, he went off to take his own shower.

It truly wasn't sense that I lacked, it was energy. I felt as if someone had turned the gravity dial all the way up. I needed a guarantee that exertion of any sort would make a difference in how I felt, otherwise, I may as well just lie there.

It is estimated that there are approximately 65 million women in America living with at least one chronic illness.

And I had joined their ranks. I'm sure you know someone who has a chronic illness. If it isn't you, then pick a handful of your friends, and one of them is ill.

These women are students trying to get through school. They are career women, working every day in spite of how they feel. They are mothers coping with being ill, while striving to care for their families. And they are women who have been ill for so long that they can't work anymore, although they'd love to be able to.

With every joint in my body aching as if I'd gone a few rounds in a boxing match, I lay curled on the sofa all day long, day after day, watching the Food Network. Delicious irony, since I could barely even eat. My whole life felt beyond my control, but what could I do about it? I was sick-and-tired of being sick-and-tired, so I did the only thing I could do; I prayed for inspiration.

I realized that everything I'd studied, everything I had learned, and all that I had experienced in my life had actually prepared me for this. I decided I wasn't going to let chronic illness write the end of my story for me. I was ready to do whatever it took to get off the couch, shed this wretched hoodie and yoga pants, and clean myself up. But, what would my first step be?

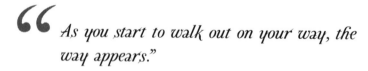

" *As you start to walk out on your way, the way appears."*

- Rumi

♥ Who could I look to for guidance or inspiration?

♥ What was I going to do about food when everything was making me sick?

♥ Would I ever feel happy and sexy again?

♥ Where would I find the energy to rebuild my life?

♥ How could I make the necessary changes and then maintain them?

Let me show you how I answered those questions and crafted my <u>Body, Mind, Spirit, and Style</u> approach to living well with chronic illness. I hope you will find something new, or stated in a new way, that inspires you to reclaim your life, too. Why settle for just sick and tired? Having a chronic illness (or two or three) doesn't have to be the end of your story either, it can be the beginning of a sexy new you!

XO Donna

PART ONE

Getting There

SECTION I

WELCOME TO THE CLUB

I was always envious of people who had a long string of letters after their names listing their degrees and affiliations. My chosen profession didn't use them. Much to my chagrin, at a recent doctor visit, I realized I now have that string of letters after my name, too. There it was, right across the top of the page the office assistant was reading from: Donna O'Klock; ET, GERD, HBP, IBS, UCTD, Sjogren's, and Raynaud's. Ah, well, the "what is" of what is.

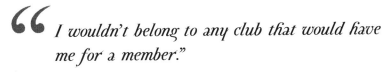

I wouldn't belong to any club that would have me for a member."

> - Groucho Marx

I love that line; it never fails to make me laugh. And now it's even funnier to me since I belong to a club I wasn't even given a choice about joining. The way I see it, the only sane choice I do have is to make the very best of it. In case you are just learning about chronic illnesses, they are loosely defined as:

- Any medical condition that lasts a year or longer.
- An illness that gets worse as time goes on.
- An illness which has symptoms that flare up occasionally.
- An illness that can be controlled, but not cured.

Approximately 65 million women in America are living with at least one chronic illness.

Our group is a diverse one, filled with every imaginable type of woman: young women trying to get through high-school or college, career women who go to their jobs every day in spite of their illness and its symptoms. Working mothers and work-at-home mothers who have to manage their family and all of its dynamics while trying to manage their own symptoms. Women who are unable to continue working, even though they'd love nothing more. Grandmothers who want to be present for their grandbabies.

These women cope with chronic illness while trying to raise and care for families, or hoping to have families one days, themselves. Approximately one-quarter of us living with chronic illness experience significant limitations in our daily activities, and most of our illnesses are not even visible to an onlooker.

As diverse as its members are, just as much diversity exists in chronic illness, which includes: Parkinson's disease, diabetes, cancer, COPD, and asthma. Chronic pain syndrome, chronic fatigue syndrome, thyroid disorders, epilepsy, Lyme disease, sickle cell anemia, and other blood and bone marrow disorders. HIV/AIDS, psoriasis, and psoriatic arthritis, chronic liver and kidney diseases. Autoimmune diseases such as multiple sclerosis, fibromyalgia, connective-tissue diseases, rheumatoid arthritis, lupus, Sjogren's syndrome, and Raynaud's disease. There are also Crohn's disease, GERD, IBS, Celiac disease and gluten-sensitivity, ulcerative colitis, and allergic reactions. Mind you, this is only a partial list.

We need to find our tribe in order to thrive.

While autoimmune diseases remain among the least understood of any illness category, I take heart because things are improving every day. For years, I felt quite alone living with ET—a rare blood/bone marrow disorder—and not having anyone but my best girlfriend, and my therapy group, to talk with about it.

If you aren't in therapy, I highly recommend it. It will add to your quality of life in ways you never imagined. Eighteen years ago, computers were slow as snails and information wasn't readily available. People tended toward privacy back then and certainly didn't talk about it if they were ill.

Over the last few years, I've seen many people in the public eye begin to speak up about living with chronic illness. Michael J. Fox was diagnosed with Parkinson's disease in the early 90's and is now the biggest advocate for more research and treatment. Toni Braxton has lupus. Halle Berry has type-1 diabetes, Tom Hanks has type-2 diabetes. Cher has had chronic fatigue syndrome since 1998. Prince had epilepsy during his childhood. Sinead O'Connor has fibromyalgia as does Morgan Freeman. Kathleen Turner has RA. And Robin Roberts of "Good Morning America" has been treated for both cancer and a bone marrow disease.

I am not alone in dealing with chronic illness, and if these people are out there fully living their lives, I can, too.

In the years since I was first diagnosed, I've seen increases in technology, improvements in pharmaceuticals, cooperation between modalities, and a growing acceptance of mind-body medicine. Not slowly and steadily, but exponentially and in unison! We now have the ability to reach out and connect with one another, sharing our experiences and finding support. And the medical community and researchers are doing the same.

Many resources are available to us; from our doctors, hospitals, clinics, and both in books and online, as well as support groups for each individual illness, and for chronic illnesses as a whole. Just like everything else on the Internet, I've found groups that are nothing more than people who want to feel sorry for themselves, and have company while doing so. I have also seen a lot of misinformation...caveat emptor. However, a lot of groups are positive and uplifting.

In his book, Outliers, Malcolm Gladwell introduced the idea that you have to practice or apprentice for 10,000 hours to become great at something. Unlike a 40-hour work week, chronic illness is a 24 hours a day, seven days a week. Allowing for eight hours sleep each night, that's 5,696 hours per year. I decided to make my life better eight years ago… so right now I have logged at least 40,000+ hours of practice. I don't know whether I am great at this yet, but I am better, much better. And working toward healing every day.

It isn't my intention to write a scholarly book; many wonderful ones have already been written. All of the suggestions and advice I offer are my own (unless otherwise noted) and were arrived at through direct experience. Some ideas are from friends also living with chronic illnesses who have generously shared their knowledge.

My best advice is not to let illness become all-consuming. Don't use your illness as an excuse for not living your life as fully as possible, or for not pursuing your dreams. Keep moving forward, no matter how slowly. There is no hurry.

Most of all, let illness be your reminder that you are precious; allow it to be the means to develop empathy and compassion for yourself. Know that your illness isn't the sum of you, it's just one part of the magnificent puzzle that makes you, you.

Our success at anything is based upon what goes on between our ears. Keep an open mind. Let yourself have fun. Don't worry about getting it right. The whole point of life is to feel good, and it is possible to not only feel good, but also to thrive in spite of living with chronic illnesses.

> *You are the community now. Be a lamp for yourselves. Be your own refuge. Seek for no other. All things must pass. Strive on diligently. Don't give up."*
>
> - Buddha

ACCEPTANCE

It is said that every good story contains a conflict. Illness creates that conflict. Like the hero in a good story, how we perceive the conflict, respond to it, and then rise above it, are what make for both an interesting read, and a soul-satisfying life.

The Conflict: We were healthy, probably happily living our lives, dreaming and making plans for our future. Suddenly, chronic illness intrudes.

Possible Scenarios: We can ignore the situation and carry on just as we were. Denial. We can feel so sorry for ourselves that we give up. We can make a bit of an effort on our own behalf, and choose to play the victim.

Or, we can commit to doing whatever it takes to manage this and feel great again!

Best Case: Acceptance. We become fully present, assess our situation, start seeing potential and even possibilities. We make a plan, rally support, and execute our plan.

Remember: our doctors can give us advice and medicine, but we have to do the work of building a healthful life ourselves.

Result: Triumph. Based on our decisive action, we have put in place a supportive network, made positive choices and created constructive habits, and built a new life designed to keep us feeling healthy, happy, and sexy.

As my friend Candy Barone, a personal coach, advises her clients, "Be your own hero!"

> **" "** *It's your road, and yours alone. Others may walk it with you, but none can walk it for you."*
>
> - Rumi

I had never had an illness that an antibiotic couldn't cure. When I became ill, I'll admit, I felt sorry for myself for a while. A long while.

And I felt stupid for wanting my old life back, and that made me angry. I damned sure wasn't going to let an illness limit me, or define me, but I was having trouble rising to my expectations of myself. It's hard to go to battle when you can't get out of bed. That was, in fact, the lesson for me. I didn't need to 'go to battle.' The only enemy to be defeated was my way of thinking.

I decided to be gentle with myself. To be patient. I trusted eventually I would figure out how to live my best life with what I had going on. And I became stronger through acceptance.

With acceptance, we can make our life the best that it can be. We can take our medicine, and we can look closely at our lifestyle to see where changes will be helpful.

We can be honest with ourselves and the doctors about our not-so-good habits and vices.

We can choose the way we look at things, and what we will focus our attention on.

We can ask our friends and family for support and encouragement.

We really can learn to love our lives, and ourselves, right now.

" *God, grant me the serenity to accept the things I cannot change,*

The courage to change the things I can,

And the wisdom to know the difference."

I know it sounds like a stretch. It's not necessarily easy to accept things we cannot change, but eventually we must, and here's why, from Tara Mohr's book, *Playing Big*:

" *It takes energy to resist what is there. Chronically pushing away your experience will lead to chronically feeling tired.*"

We're already there, we are feeling sick and tired. But we will have more energy when we aren't resistant. By embracing what's going on, and by accepting what is, you learn to embrace yourself and grow in ways you never thought possible.

> " *Acceptance of one's life has nothing to do with resignation; it does not mean running away from the struggle. On the contrary, it means accepting it as it comes, with all the handicaps of heredity, of suffering, of psychological complexes and injustices."*

- Paul Tournier

BOTTOM LINE:

Acceptance just feels better, lighter, and it's a way of spiraling upward. It offers potential, like the chlorophyll-infused leaves and buds in springtime, it's full of promise. Resignation is always a downward spiral. Choose light by choosing to accept.

BEFORE AND AFTER

People often deny what's happening, or what will happen, because of a tendency to think life was better before we became ill. It's all some people ever talk about.

But to live life that way, focusing on the past, is to live as if everything wonderful has already happened. That is dying to the future. And who says our "after" has to be worse?

I'm living my "after," and I can honestly say my life is better in many ways than before I developed these illnesses. I am an evolving work-in-progress, and I see that as a good thing.

In the last few years I've come to accept the wholeness of who I am. I make it a point to enjoy what I do. I dream about where I intend to go, what I want to accomplish, and illness doesn't hinder any of that.

How did I get here? Acceptance.

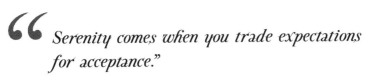 *Serenity comes when you trade expectations for acceptance."*

         - Buddha

As adults, we generally know what's in our best interest and what isn't, yet we often test the limits. Like a high-stakes game of Hold 'Em poker, when you live with chronic illness, you're always "all in." How you play the hand you've been dealt is going to make all the difference in the quality of your life. You may not like your hand, but ignoring it won't change it. The prize for playing the hand you've got is living a full life and feeling good as you do it.

To win that prize you may be required to accept an awful lot of things:

- ♥ Your diet may need to change in order to become well-balanced and nutritious.

- ♥ You may need to follow specific food guidelines which will allow your body to perform at its best.

- ♥ You may need to exercise, especially if it's something you've avoided or never done.

- ♥ Taking some quiet-time for daily meditation or prayer, even just 10 minutes, will be helpful

- ♥ You need to sleep more (8 to 9 hours is best) and rest during the day.

- ♥ You may need to drink more water, and give up artificial sweeteners and diet drinks.

- ♥ Or give up wheat, dairy, eggs, nuts, chocolate, sugar

- ♥ You may need to minimize your alcohol consumption.

- ♥ and, of course, stop smoking.

None of this is easy at first. Years ago, after becoming ill and being in group therapy for a while, my therapist suggested I stop drinking for a couple of months to "see what came up." My doctors had told me I could have wine or a margarita because it was probably helpful in easing my anxiety. But she wanted to see what it was that was making me anxious. I glibly agreed to either four or six months. I don't remember which.

Unfortunately, I made this commitment right before the holidays. Bad timing for me, or perhaps she planned it this way, but in either case, I found myself standing in the wine aisle of the grocery store at Thanksgiving having a meltdown. I was looking at all the delicious wines and champagnes I couldn't have, thinking of all the parties I wouldn't attend, and crying openly in front of other customers. You could say I was having a lot of trouble accepting something I couldn't change.

That was when I learned the Serenity Prayer. I learned to take things one day at a time, and I learned that acceptance is generally the sanest option. Recently, I heard Pico Ayer, world-traveler and novelist, say,

> " *If I really want to change my life, I might best begin by changing my mind.*"

Once I have accepted something, I figure out how to have fun with it. I change my thinking from feeling deprived or limited, to feeling challenged and inspired. Changing our minds about what it means to live a life that includes chronic illness is our biggest challenge.

What can we learn from it? How can we grow? How do we become happier and more fulfilled in spite of it, or maybe even because of it?

For myself, I found illness gave me a renewed sense of purpose and focus. For the first time in my life, I realized I didn't have all the time in the world. Not in the abstract, but concretely, as in I could die much sooner than I ever thought.

Illness can rekindle a dream that has been patiently waiting for us to return. It can inspire us to become someone we've always wanted to be. Ultimately, it can lead us to where our personal strength and power will be found.

And in my book, that's all pretty darned sexy.

BE HERE NOW

" *The secret of health for both mind and body is not to mourn for the past, nor to worry about the future, but to live in the present moment wisely and earnestly."*

- Buddha

Occasionally, I catch myself dwelling on the past, thinking about my life before I developed these illnesses. I had more energy, I looked and felt more fit, and I believed I had all the time in the world to do everything that I wanted.

When I get lost daydreaming wistfully about the past, remembering these three words always brings me back to the present: Be. Here. Now.

You've all heard these words, so how about a little backstory?

In the 1960's, Richard Alpert and his friend Timothy Leary, both psychologists at Harvard University, were caught experimenting with psychedelics. Consequently, and quite understandably, they were both fired. Richard Alpert, disappointed because all of their research into the therapeutic effects of psychedelic drugs (particularly LSD) hadn't helped him resolve his spiritual questions, left America on a sojourn to India, leaving everything behind. Timothy Leary went on to write and speak, promoting hallucinogens as a way of encouraging people to become sensitive to their levels of consciousness by going within. He influenced many musicians, authors, and performers.

The counter-culture phrase born of this experimentation was: Turn on. Tune in. Drop out.

When Richard Alpert returned to America a changed man in 1971, he wrote a book about his experiences in India entitled *Remember, Be Here Now*. It chronicled his metaphysical, spiritual, and religious changes, and his relationship with his guru, who had renamed him Baba Ram Dass, or "servant of god."

All of this was exceptional back then; nobody was meditating or doing yoga. Nobody from the West, especially a non-Hindu, had ever studied with an Eastern teacher before and had a guru-student relationship. What he learned and shared paved the way for so many things that are an everyday part of our lives now.

I remember what a groundbreaker this book was; for a while it was the most popular book in English. It was the first guide on spirituality, yoga and meditation. *Remember, Be Here Now* became a counterculture bible-of-sorts for a generation of people, myself included, who were hungry for transformation.

Through the years, Ram Dass' teachings have influenced many writers, thinkers, thought-leaders, teachers, and yoga aficionados. Among the most familiar to us are Dr. Wayne Dyer, George Harrison of The Beatles, Michael Crichton, author of *Jurassic Park*, and Steve Jobs of Apple. As I wrote this, I realized they are all gone now.

Ram Dass continues to leave his mark on the world by writing more books and by teaching and promoting loving-service, harmonious-business practices, and conscious-care for the dying, which is where hospice care came from.

Why is all of this important?

Because we have a natural tendency to break our lives into two parts: the part Before we became ill, and the part Afterward.

I've realized nothing can be gained by dwelling on the past and thinking it was better. Just as there is no point in all of the "what ifs?" of the future.

Watching one of Oprah's Super Soul Sunday programs, her guest was someone I'd never heard of, her friend Bishop Jakes. What he said resonated for me.

❝ *When you hold on to your history, you do it at the expense of your destiny."*

Being here now gives us the power to direct our thoughts and live our lives in the present moment.

PRACTICE MAKES PERFECT

It's certainly easy to get caught up in feeling bad; you have another headache, or even worse, a migraine. You awakened feeling nauseated again. You can't close your hand around your coffee cup. And to add insult to injury, you can't even get the damned child-proof cap on your meds opened. You're running late for work, but can't leave the bathroom just yet.

Some days, you get up and shower, blow your hair dry, then sit down and cry because you've run out of energy. You wonder how you will make it to the end of the day, right?

In recovery groups one of the principle foundations is taking things one day at a time. Just today.

If today seems too long to deal with, take it one hour at a time. This hour.

And if 60 minutes seems interminably long, just think about the next few minutes. Right now.

There have been days I've walked around singing the Doobie Brothers song, "Minute, by minute, by minute, by minute, I keep holding on."

When life is the pits, it's normal to space-out or daydream. And although people spend almost half of their awake time thinking about something besides what they're doing, ironically, daydreaming doesn't usually make them happy.

The greater our ability to pay attention, the happier we are. Some religions suggest happiness can be found by focusing on what's happening at the moment, or being here now."

Those three words again: Be. Here. Now.

> *It is the familiar that eludes us in life. What is before our nose is what we see last."*
>
> - William Barrett

When the migraines first began that are one of the hallmarks of the blood disorder I have, I was frightened. They would crescendo into a nauseating lightshow which left me with a stiff neck, and weighted down, feeling as if I were wearing a dentist's lead apron. I began to dread every little flicker of light, worrying that I would get another migraine. It was obvious to me that I needed to find a way to work through this, rather than living in fear.

One day as a migraine developed, I decided to play it cool and see what happened. Everything unfolded just as always, but this time my curiosity allowed me to make note of the order and duration of the lightshow, and to observe the pulsating, neon-bright colors of the electric serpent which is the star of the show.

I focused on breathing fully, and when the lightshow ended twenty minutes later, my body relaxed. This time I didn't feel wiped out by the experience. Perhaps becoming anxious is like trying to put out a fire with gasoline?

Learning to stay present takes practice, but mindfulness can be learned. Stay with what's happening by calling forth as much curiosity as you can muster. Here are some ideas on how to Be Here Now:

1) Practice noticing yourself as you go about your day.

This is me blowing my hair dry.

This is me walking to the kitchen to get a glass of water.

This is me eating breakfast.

This is me driving to work, grateful to have this time to sit down.

This is me talking to a friend/employee/co-worker.

This is me cooking dinner. Or playing with the children, or with my pet.

This is me sitting in this comfortable chair, drinking this cup of tea.

Notice how you are sitting. Are your legs under you? Are they crossed?

Mine were crossed at my knee as I wrote this, and I just uncrossed them. Now I feel my bare feet on the tile floor, and I can also feel that I need to sweep it.

2) Practice paying attention to feelings and sounds outside of yourself.

If the air-conditioner/heater is running, do you hear it?

Do you feel it on your skin?

What do you hear outside your room? Traffic? Children playing? Dogs barking? Quiet?

What do you hear inside the room? Inside the house?

Is there a scent in your house? Do you like it?

How does your home look? Pleasant? Chaotic?

Is there something you've been trying to ignore?

What do you see outside your windows?

Is there anything you never noticed before?

3) Practice turning inward, with a sense of curiosity and exploration.

Close your eyes for a minute and think about what is going on.

What are you feeling?

Notice all of your feelings and thoughts, don't push any away.

Where do you feel them? In your gut? In your back or shoulders?

Are all of the thoughts true?

Are you breathing fully or holding your breath?

Is there anything you can do to resolve this?

If it can't be resolved right now, can you just sit with it? Are you willing?

When it's your choice to stay present, does that make it easier?

4) When all else fails, do something.

Wash dishes. Make the bed. Fold the laundry. Iron clothes. Bake a batch of cookies, with or without gluten. Vacuum the rug. Sweep the floor. Do some mending. Balance your checkbook. Water the plants. Pet your cat or dog. Paint your toenails. Paint someone else's toenails. Brush their hair. Massage their shoulders. Ask them to massage yours. Curl up and read a book. Read a story aloud. Sing along with the radio or a CD. Dance around the living room. Go out for a walk, even in the rain. Call a friend and ask them how they are and be present for them.

Do these as wholeheartedly for as long as you can. You will feel better, I promise.

" *While washing the dishes one should only be washing the dishes, which means that while washing the dishes one should be completely aware of the fact that one is washing the dishes. At first glance, that might seem a little silly: why put so much stress on a simple thing? But that's precisely the point. The fact that I am standing there and washing these bowls is a wondrous reality. I'm being completely myself, following my breath, conscious of my presence, and conscious of my thoughts and actions. There's no way I can be tossed around mindlessly like a bottle slapped here and there on the waves."*

- Thich Nhat Hanh

ALL YOU NEED IS LOVE

I recently reread Julia Cameron's exquisite book, *The Artist's Way*. In it she wrote about experiencing the end of a love affair which she said left her mute and ashamed. She received a letter from her (obviously very dear and very wise) friend Laura:

> **"** *Just a quick note to say – do not chide yourself, berate yourself, belittle yourself for having fallen in love with someone who did not receive your love with the care and grace it deserves… just don't beat yourself up for having loved."*

Beautiful advice, and as I read it I thought, what if I were to change the subject from love to illness? What then?

> **"** *Just a quick note to say – do not chide yourself, berate yourself, belittle yourself for having fallen ill. Love yourself with the care*

and grace you deserve . . . just don't beat yourself up for being ill."

What a difference it would have made if I had remembered those words years ago. Beating ourselves up looking for an explanation, or somewhere to lay blame, when we fall ill is an easy hell to fall into. Surely an outside reason, a cause, must be responsible. Or something I did, or didn't do.

Finding none, I took it personally and felt singled-out. And angry. Eventually I realized my attitude made me feel worse physically, too. When I finally began treating myself more gently, I felt better.

❝ *You were born with wings. You are not meant to crawl, so don't. You have wings, learn to use them and fly."*

- Rumi

Illness disrupts our plans and changes our direction. Before illness there seemed to be so many places to go and things we could do. Now we often focus on feeling stuck, and the longer we stay there; feeling stuck, angry, or victimized, the more likely we are to give up.

We start owning the illness. "My diabetes," you say. "My arthritis," or "My damned thyroid disease."

Once you let illness move in and make itself comfortable, it expands and takes up the space where joy and possibility used to live.

Owning an illness by calling it mine, "my whatever," minimizes the possibility that one day I won't have it anymore.

I prefer to think of it as a temporary aspect of myself; the blood disease or the auto-immune disorder. Thinking this way inspires me to treat myself as lovingly and compassionately as I can. By doing so, I put myself in the best position to make my healing possible.

> **"** *You, yourself, as much as anybody else in the entire Universe, deserve your love and affection."*
>
> - Buddha

Illness is a journey we ultimately must take on our own. It is an inner journey, although outwardly many others are involved: the doctors and nurses who treat us, the pharmacist who dispenses the medicines we take to control our symptoms, our family and friends who care about us and for us.

Still, we walk our path alone, and it can become a magnificent growth opportunity. Illness can be a chance to heal our mind and spirit, which will have a positive impact on our body and on our lives.

Fill yourself up with love and gratitude for all that you are, even for this journey that you're on, and for all of the unknown opportunities that lie ahead of you. Being your own hero starts with loving yourself.

> **"** *To love oneself is the beginning of a lifelong romance."*
>
> - Oscar Wilde

I had lived well with the blood disorder for nine or ten years, when I was also diagnosed with autoimmune disorders. It took a while for me to see the metaphor and the irony: my immune system had begun working overtime, attacking my healthy body tissue.

Small wonder, since I had been attacking myself the majority of my life: I had always been critical of myself and my unique ideas and way of looking at things. I worried I didn't fit in, or wasn't attractive enough, good enough, or loveable enough. Now, I had a disease to pick on me, too!

I wondered - if I learn to love and accept myself, could it have an impact on these illnesses?

I now believe that becoming ill accelerated my growth process, and is facilitating my inner-healing. As I learn to love myself, I am more open to love in general, and more able to give love freely. I am more accepting of myself and others.

Heaven knows, I'm not a saint (wouldn't want to be) and I still have a journey ahead of me to feel healthy the way I want to, both spiritually and physically. But, as I follow this path toward love, I find I am taking fewer medicines and have been able to reduce the doses of many of the drugs I take. I feel healthier and more positive now.

We all know what loving another person, or a dear pet looks like, but what does loving ourselves look like?

I demonstrate my love for myself by taking great care of myself: I eat delicious and nutritious foods. I make sure to drink enough water. I take my meds on time. I get enough sleep. I move my body regularly by doing yoga, or Nia, or going to the gym, or taking a walk outdoors in the fresh air.

I stay inspired by being curious about the world and the positive people in it. I stay focused on my dreams and goals. I listen to guided meditations and spend a few minutes every day seeking inspiration. I avoid negativity.

Every day when I wake up I can choose to love myself, and to give it my best effort, warts and all. Since I have been doing that, I've found that there's much more to love. And so much more love to give.

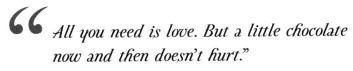 *All you need is love. But a little chocolate now and then doesn't hurt."*

- Charles Schulz

FOR THINGS TO CHANGE

I attended my first personal growth workshop, an INSIGHT Seminar, when I was in my mid-30s. Walking into the auditorium on the first day of the workshop, I was stunned by the message on a huge banner hanging above the podium:

"FOR THINGS TO CHANGE. . . FIRST I MUST CHANGE"

I had never, ever, thought about that before. Up until that moment, I thought I had no control or influence over anything that happened. I didn't realize the connection between the act of changing myself and its impact on what was happening around me.

Now I know I am accountable for my life and what's going on in it. I have influence on what occurs in my life. I can create/co-create how my life works, and what is included in it, and what is excluded from it.

Change is the only constant there is, and I've learned from experience that willingness to change, or adaptability, is the key to living well, and especially living well with chronic illness.

Up until I became ill, I had done everything "right" for the majority of my life. My only indulgence was frozen margaritas with a deliciously salted rim.

- ♥ I ate well: fresh food cooked from scratch at home, home-made whole wheat bread, a knowledgeable and expansive vegetarian diet and I only rarely indulged in packaged food like crackers or pasta.
- ♥ I exercised four to five times a week because I loved it.

- ♥   I drank lots of water and herbal teas.
- ♥   I slept like a baby, for a solid 8-9 hours each night.
- ♥   I loved my work and looked forward to each day.
- ♥   I had a small but solid community of like-minded friends that I enjoyed.
- ♥   I had a great relationship with my son and my extended family.

I couldn't have been more shocked when I found out the psychedelic migraines I was having were caused by a blood disorder. How could this have happened me?

That sentiment was echoed by all of my friends. "Jeez, you're the healthiest person we know! How could this have happened to you?"

That's just one of the oddities of being a human. Bad things do happen. How we learn to view them, deal with them, and move beyond them can give us a great quality of life, or just merely an existence.

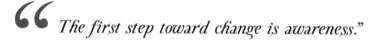

" *The first step toward change is awareness."*

– Nataniel Branden

Since you have picked up this book, I assume you are living with a chronic illness, or two or three, and you are not satisfied with the direction your life has taken because of it. And I'll bet that you feel sick and tired, but you're not feeling very sexy.

I understand. I wish I could tell you I found an easy solution so that our lives will be blissful in spite of everything, but chronic illness isn't that way.

Here's the good news - you have the ability to make of your life exactly what you want, but you may have to make some changes to get yourself to that place.

"For things to change, FIRST I must change."

Make this your mantra. Believe in it. Trust it. Nothing can change in our lives until we change our mind, our attitude, our belief system, or our habits.

What if you hate change? What if you're thinking that change isn't fun or easy, how do you know it will it be worth it?

Let me answer those questions with a question of my own: Who promised us life would be easy? But can it be much more difficult than it is right now?

Not everything will be fun; some things in life just aren't. But many things certainly will be, and if we change how we approach them, we can make them fun.

As far as change being easy, it's not hard. Will it be worth it? For the chance to feel better, yes. For the chance to feel better about yourself, absolutely. Knowing you can affect positive change in your life is outright empowering!

The changes I present for you to explore can not only provide a better quality of life, but can also have a positive impact on the people around you: your family, your life-partners, your friends, the people you work with, and those you meet. You will become a role model, someone who helps others see it is possible to change and become happier. We can become the best version of ourselves and live beautiful, fulfilling lives even while living with chronic illness.

But the other thing to remember will act as your oars, steering you:

"Take care of YOURSELF first, in order to take care of others."

This cardinal rule covers all areas of your life: physical, mental, and spiritual, and here is where we begin our journey: by putting ourselves first. You first. Before your kids, your partner, your friends, your extended family, and the people you work with.

But isn't it SELFISH to put myself first? No. Contrary to what our parents, teachers, society, religious institutions, and authority-figures-in-general have taught you, putting yourself first is not selfish.

The definition of "selfish" is: Lacking consideration for others. Excessive or exclusive concern with oneself, and without regard for others.

If you only put yourself first, you'd be selfish. However, I learned that you put yourself first in order to take care of others. Think about this for a minute, you're of no use to anyone if you're sick all of the time, or dead, because you didn't take care of yourself. Drastic example, I know, but the point needs to be made.

On an airplane, you are always told to put your mask on FIRST, then help the others around you. You still have the responsibility to consider others and their needs.

But if you don't take care of yourself, who will? Sacrifice is not the same as being generous. And when you're living with chronic illness, or any kind of illness for that matter, sacrifice only makes you a martyr. And we know how that usually ends, don't we?

You are of little use to anyone else, and you aren't a very good role model either, if you are too sick to be present because you didn't put your needs first. It's all right to set limits and have clear boundaries. Actually, it's absolutely necessary, in order to raise children who won't grow up to be selfish themselves, always expecting their needs to be met immediately.

It's all right to say, "No. I can't do that today," without apologizing or explaining to anyone. Demonstrate what taking good care of yourself looks like to those around you. Learn what you need in order to feel well. Then learn to give yourself exactly what you need.

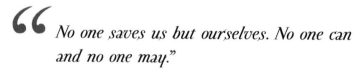

" *No one saves us but ourselves. No one can and no one may.*"

- Buddha

This may be a very big change for you, depending on your age. As women, we were often raised to take care of everyone else first, even at the expense of our own needs. We were praised for being selfless, told we were being generous, and given lots of approval.

My mother was very loving and warm, but she had some funny ideas about what was selfish and what wasn't. Even when she fell ill, she still felt obligated to take care of everyone else, rather than ask anyone to take care of her. She never realized we would have jumped at the chance to do anything for her.

As children, it would have taught us to consider other's needs and allowed us to contribute, even at an early age. She also had some funny ideas about what you had to accept in life. She believed you had to settle for whatever you got and be grateful you got anything at all.

But what if you needed or preferred something else?

I know the answer now: it is our responsibility to see that our needs are met. Nobody else can do this for us. Expecting anyone to read your mind, or thinking that if someone loved you, they would know what you needed, is co-dependent. The best thing you can do for yourself, your family, and your friends is to ask for exactly what you want, and take care of yourself first so you can be there for them.

How do you take care of yourself first? What would that look like? Here are some examples:

1. You really need to lie down now. But the dishes, the laundry, preparing dinner, or a family member wants your attention. Do you give up on lying down?
   No. Announce you are going to lie down for 30 minutes, and you will sort things out when that time is up. Then do it. Go lie down. Unless there's an emergency, everything will still be there waiting for you in 30 minutes and you'll feel more able to give what's needed.

2. You've realized, in order to feel better, you need to make healthy changes to your diet. Actually, to everyone's diet. Do you just impose it on your family?
   No. First you tell everyone you are all going to eat better starting next week. Then ease into it.

To make it easier on yourself, don't take the kids to the grocery store with you. Not only do you have to shop when you are sick and tired, but also to manage their expectations as well, and they want everything they see on TV. Remember - you are the parent, the responsible adult. You are in charge.

3. If you need to eat at certain times in order to manage your medicines and how they make you feel, set the time that works for you and stick to it. Create structure around meals: no skipping meals or eating the kids' leftovers, or grazing all day. Nutritious meals at regular intervals are what it takes to feel better and maintain a healthy weight.

4. You need to go to bed earlier in order to get enough rest. Do it. Keep your commitment to yourself. When you are chronically ill, routine is your support system and maintaining a schedule will help you feel more in control, which is a gift in itself. If your children aren't on a schedule, now is the time. Routine is better for children, too.

5. If you need to say "No" to things, just do it. Practice saying this, "No, that won't work for me." If something else will work, then offer that option. No need to explain or apologize. And from this day forward, don't use your illness as an excuse for not doing something you don't want to do. I used to do that because I didn't have good boundaries. And I was afraid the other person would think I was selfish.

6. If you don't feel well enough on a given day to do everything you said you would, renegotiate the things you can. Apologize and let them know you may feel well enough at a later date, but today you cannot do what you said you would. In this case, your illness is your reason, not your excuse.

7. Oh, what a can of worms family gatherings can be, but it's really this simple: if you don't feel well enough to make an event, don't go. If you don't feel well enough to host an event, just say so. Setting healthy boundaries with our family can be a big change, and a big challenge, and there may be some pushback. Stand your ground. People may be disappointed, including you, but these people are supposed to love you the most, and they should want what is best for you.

> **"** *If being disappointed is the worst thing that ever happens to me, I'm good with that."*
>
> Donna O'Klock

8. Parties, meetings, happy hours, friend's events - all the same as above. If you don't feel well enough to make it, don't go and don't worry. Stay home and take care of yourself. I've missed many special events I was looking forward to: Thanksgiving dinners, nights out with friends, Christmas parties, motorcycle rides, a Raul Malo & The Mavericks concert. Of course, I was disappointed at the time, but honestly, I wouldn't have had any fun if I had forced myself to go. I got to hear all about it later and saw photos on Facebook the next day. Not the same, I know, but at least I was at home in bed and comfortable. Other great things will appear in my life, as I know will in yours!

Your mission is to learn how to take the best possible care of yourself, and with that comes a critical change in your thinking; you must learn to take care of yourself first, in order to take care of others. Remember, it's not selfish, unless it is, and you will know the difference. Your health right now may be critical enough that you have to make yourself a priority so that you can stay alive. Whatever the reason, put yourself first. You are doing this so that you can be present for the people in your life that you love, for your friends, and for your life's work. You're valuable, and you're worth it.

AN ATTITUDE OF GRATITUDE

Ever since I woke up this morning and made the bed, all I've wanted to do is crawl right back into it. I feel as if someone unplugged me. I made myself a cup of coffee, disappointed I was out of cream. I compensated by barely scalding some milk and adding it to my coffee with a little bit of honey. It was delicious, so I got over my disappointment and gratefully sipped it while I wrote my morning pages.

When I finished them, I wrote a thank you note to my boss for a book he had given me as a gift a few weeks ago. I have been reading it at bedtime each night. I thanked him for his generosity, told him again how happy I was to be working at his salon. I even went as far as to tell him I thought he was my "guardian angel."

I felt silly, and wondered whether to tear it up and write a new note. Now I am glad I risked looking foolish by saying that, since he passed away soon after.

> **"** *Gratitude is the single most important ingredient to living a successful and fulfilled life."*
>
> - Jack Canfield

The book my boss gave me was *The Complete Works* by Florence Scovel Shinn. Published in 1925, it's a compilation about "The Law of Attraction."

Her ideas were ahead of their time, and may still be considered so by some, but they opened the door for personal growth. She taught us we are magnets, and we have the power to attract both consciously and unconsciously. Her books also taught that being grateful is the way to help us create prosperity, solve problems, and have better health.

I'm sure you are familiar with some of these inspiring teachers and thought-leaders: Buddha, Rumi, Zig Ziglar, Dr. Wayne Dyer, Deepak Chopra, Dale Carnegie, Jack Canfield, Julia Cameron, Marianne Williamson, The Dalai Lama, Pema Chodron. One teaching they all have in common: **GRATITUDE**.

Being grateful for things in your life is indeed magnetic, and as the infomercials always say, "but wait, there's more!" Staying focused and grateful for what I have in my life has made me happier, more relaxed, and more comfortable.

I wondered if my happiness was just a coincidence, or if it was because I paid less attention to what I was unhappy about? As it turns out, there are three biochemical reasons gratitude makes us happier: dopamine, serotonin, and oxytocin. Dopamine and serotonin are linked to being happy and to pleasant emotions. Oxytocin is closely associated with love and bonding.

Practicing gratitude boosts the neurotransmitter dopamine, which affects the part of our brain involved in motivation, reward, and pleasure. Consciously being grateful toward other people increases the activity in our "social dopamine circuits," and makes interacting with others much more enjoyable.

Another effect of practicing gratitude is that it increases our body's serotonin by engaging the parasympathetic nervous system and producing feelings of peacefulness and calmness. These positive feelings benefit your heart, which helps your cardiovascular system function efficiently.

And, last but not least, the hormone oxytocin is central to physical bonding. Our oxytocin levels rise dramatically when we hug someone we love, or have sex, or breast-feed our babies. Oxytocin adds to our feelings of belonging and being part of a community.

Thinking about the things in our lives we have to be grateful for causes us to focus on the positive things happening in our life. This increases our dopamine, serotonin, and oxytocin levels, naturally causing an upward spiral of happiness!

> " *Everything is interconnected. Gratitude improves sleep. Sleep reduces pain. Reduced pain improves your mood. Improved mood reduces anxiety, which improves focus and planning. Focus and planning help with decision-making. Decision-making further reduces anxiety and improves enjoyment. Enjoyment gives you more to be grateful for, which keeps that loop of the upward spiral going. Enjoyment also makes it more likely that you'll exercise and be social, which, in turn, will make you happier.*"
>
> - Eric Barker

WHERE TO BEGIN

It may seem hard to find anything to be grateful for when you live with chronic illness. It's probably become commonplace to feel exhausted, uncomfortable, or in pain.

Our medicines, despite being either lifesaving or beneficial, aren't without their added side effects. Being unable to go out and socialize the way we once did can leave us feeling dejected, left out, or downright lonely. All the more reason to develop an attitude of gratitude.

I longed to have my old life back for a while, before I finally decided to take stock of everything good in my life:

- ♥ I have satisfying work.
- ♥ I have pursuits/hobbies I'm passionate about.
- ♥ I enjoy my co-workers.
- ♥ I had a beautiful drive to work.
- ♥ I had a great place to work.
- ♥ I have a sweet son to love.
- ♥ And a life-partner I love.
- ♥ I have family, and extended family, to love.
- ♥ I have friends who inspire me.
- ♥ I have medicines that keep me alive.
- ♥ I enjoy learning and being creative.
- ♥ I love to cook, read, travel, and take photos, and I am able do all of that.
- ♥ I have food to eat.
- ♥ I have a roof over my head, a bed to sleep in, and hot running water.
- ♥ I have a computer, and I have books, I have pens and paper.
- ♥ I could easily go on and on.

Thinking about what I was grateful for in my life showed me that when we look for things to be grateful for, we will find them. I could have continued my gratitude exercise to include my city, my state, my country, the planet.

The opposite is true, too; when you look for what's wrong in your life, or in other people, or out in the world, you will find it. The question becomes: which do you want to focus on?

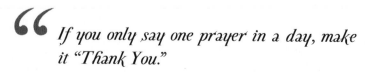

If you only say one prayer in a day, make it "Thank You."

- Rumi

Along with gratitude, I practice focusing on my intentions, what I intend to do and create in my life. When you take a motorcycle safety class to become a better rider, one of the first things they teach you is don't look where you don't want to go. It's a given that if you focus on the pothole in the road ahead, you will undoubtedly hit it.

To frame this more positively, look in the direction you do want to go, don't fixate on the difficulties that might lie ahead. Florence Scovel-Shinn called this, "The Law of Increase," and it stated: "What you focus on, you will get more of."

What do I want more of in my life? That's where our focus should be.

Most of us are crystal clear on what we don't want in our lives, but although we know that, nothing seems to change. That's because there are two things at play here: we are focusing on what we don't want, and we may lack clarity about exactly what we do want.

Based on Scovel's "Law of Increase," if we always focus on what we don't want and how we don't want to feel, we'll continue to have what we don't want, and feel the way we don't want to feel. Can you see where it would be beneficial to shift where we place our attention?

Begin to focus on what you DO want to have in your life, and how you DO want to feel. Don't worry about how it will happen, and don't let your ideas of reality get in the way of imagining what you desire.

Next, imagine how you will feel when you get what you want. The more real the feeling becomes; the better it is for you.

I take a few minutes each day to sit quietly and focus on what I want in my life. I envision I already have it, feel my joy about it, and psych myself up to where I'm grinning like the Cheshire Cat. When I reach that heartfelt grin, I know I've done my part. By focusing, I've set my intention.

I often do this in my gratitude writing, too. I focus on how thankful I am for something as if I already have it. For example, "I am grateful I have so much energy today!" or "I am grateful my back and shoulders feel so relaxed today."

To help you get started, I have included Gratitude Exercises on the following page. No matter what you come up with, it's a great place and a great time to get started. You can't do it wrong.

I hope writing Gratitudes becomes a practice that includes a lovely reward or a cup of tea afterward. Focusing on a gratitude practice can be a reflective time to share with your partner or even your children. What a nice practice to teach them when they're young. You can use it as an opportunity to sit quietly, or listen to music, as you focus on everything you do have and are grateful for.

If you can truly find nothing for which to be grateful, please don't give up. Put it away and try again the next day. Just find ONE thing and write it down. Do it again the next day.

Gratitude is magnetic. The more things you find, the more you will attract. When we focus on the positive in our lives, we attract positive people, positive situations, and positive results. Because of all of this, gratitude is now the attitude I choose to maintain.

Gratitude Exercises

How to: As you think about the headings in the Column A, make your list. First thought, no need to censor, just get those things off your chest. You can always do longer lists if you want to, just grab a sheet of blank paper. Let it all out, and remember - this is for your eyes only. You can't do it wrong. When you've finished Column A, move on to Column B.

Column A

Things that I don't want. Things I am unhappy about. Things I don't like, or I hate.

Column B

I'd rather have... I'd love... I want...

1.

2.

3.

4.

5.

6.

7.

8.

9.

Now, for each corresponding number above, write down something you'd prefer in **Column B**. For example: If column A1. had, "I hate feeling sick and tired all of the time," In B1. I would write, "I'd love to feel sexy and energetic instead."

What would you prefer? What would bring you joy? What do you dream of, or long for? No matter how trivial or unrealistic it may seem to you, write it down. As I said, first thought, no limits!

Here's the last part, and this is how we create more of what exactly we want in our lives: by acknowledging it is in our lives right now, and being grateful for it. The more gratitude we can muster, the more we have of those things we want!

How to: Take each of your preferences from Column B and write each below next to its corresponding number in a sentence that expresses your gratitude for all of this which you already possess. Trust me, you do.

This is where everything comes together: my original sentence in Column A1. was, "I hate feeling sick and tired all of the time." It became, "I'd love to feel sexy and energetic," in Column B1. because that's what I'd rather have.

Now I am going to write: *"I'm grateful for the sexiness and energy I do have."*

I'm grateful for:

1. I am grateful for the _____
   that I do have.

2. I am grateful for the _____
   that I do have.

3. I am grateful for the _____
   that I do have.

4. I am grateful for the _____
   that I do have.

5. I am grateful for the _____
   that I do have.

6. I am grateful for the _____
   that I do have.

7. I am grateful for the _____
   that I do have.

8. I am grateful for the _____
   that I do have.

9. I am grateful for the _____
   that I do have.

There you go, you are well on our way. Any time you find yourself feeling down or overwhelmed, sit down and start with what's going on that you don't like. Move on to what you'd rather have, then be grateful for how much of it you already have.

Eventually, you may want to make this a daily practice. Expressing our gratitude before bedtime seems to be particularly powerful. Buy yourself a blank journal just for writing your gratitudes. It can be as simple, or as elegant as you like. I surprised myself when I recently bought a new Gratitude Journal in pink. Pink... I've never been a pink girl, and now I can't get enough of it!

Over time you will notice many of the things that you disliked in your life have either diminished, or disappeared altogether. Things that you love and are grateful for will blossom. And you'll notice how well you feel more of the time.

Gratitude, as Martha Stewart would say, "It's a good thing."

SECTION 2

& sexy

MAKE YOUR BED

I love my bed. Everything about it, from the simple duvet and shams I bought for it, to the good night's sleep it affords me.

On days like today, with a busy week at work and too many commitments on my day off, all I want to do is crawl right back into it the minute I've crawled out of it.

To crawl back into bed as often as I want would be a kind of death. A giving up. Since it eliminates the possibility of accomplishing anything, better to leave it as a longing to be satisfied when bedtime arrives.

Granted, some days we're not well, and staying in bed is certainly the prudent thing to do. But for me, sleeping more does not necessarily equal having more energy. Have you noticed the same thing? Since my tiredness won't be satisfied, I get up, make my bed, and get moving. And keep moving.

From experience, I know I'll be fine.

WHAT'S THE POINT?

When I tell people about making my bed first thing every day, they always ask, "What's the point? You could lie back down, so why bother?" Of course I could if I wanted to, but I wouldn't.

Whether it's a function of my upbringing, or my own stubbornness, it's off-limits once it's made. My father had a military background and was an interior designer. We were taught that once your "bunk was in order, it wasn't to be disturbed until bedtime." He liked things to look good. They were a product of his design, after all. Like him, I enjoy a well-made bed in a tidy room, and I feel better because of it.

Some studies show that in order to sleep better (always a good thing when living with chronic illness), your bedroom should only be used for sleep and sex. Not working, or hanging out watching TV. Our brain should associate our bed with rest and romance, and we should create a peaceful, romantic environment conducive to both. The study said nothing about reading in bed, so I'm going to keep doing that.

I really felt validated in my bed-making habit when I heard Naval Admiral William H. McRaven's commencement speech to the 2014 graduating class at The University of Texas in Austin, his alma mater. A Navy Seal for 36 years, among the many things he spoke of, he shared this simple lesson and its importance to him:

> *If you make your bed every morning you will have accomplished the first task of the day. It will give you a small sense of pride and it will encourage you to do another task, and another, and another. [Making your bed] will also reinforce the fact that little things in life matter. And, if by chance you are having a miserable day, you will come home to a bed that is made, that you made, and it gives you encouragement that tomorrow will be better."*

I was convinced I was on to something special when I read the post, "Make Your Bed! For Productivity, Profit and Peace" in the Apartment Therapy blog. I'm a fan of productivity, profit, and especially of peace. The writer admitted he hated making his bed, reasoning that he was only going to get back into it later. When he read an excerpt from Charles Duhigg's book, *The Power of Habit*, he changed his mind. Mr. Duhigg writes that making your bed every morning is correlated with better productivity. How can doing something so quick and easy (*seriously, it takes 5 minutes*) make such a difference in your life?

The act of making your bed is one way of developing a "Keystone Habit." These are feel-good tasks, like exercising and cooking nutritious food for yourself, that can become habits and then spill over into other areas of your life. According to Mr. Duhigg, "changing, or developing, keystone habits will help other habits flourish. Essentially, a keystone habit is a catalyst for other beneficial behaviors."

Gretchen Rubin, the *New York Times* bestselling author of *The Happiness Project*, notes that, to her astonishment, when she asks people what has made a big difference in their happiness, many people cite the modest principle of 'Make Your Bed.'

Karen Miller is a wife, a mother, a Zen priest, and the author of *Hand Wash Cold* and *Momma Zen*. She believes the state of your bed represents the state of your head. I've always thought our surroundings were a reflection of how we felt about ourselves, but had never heard anyone else say it aloud.

So, why does making your bed boost happiness so effectively?

- ♥ First: it's a simple step that's quick and easy, yet makes a big difference. Everything looks neater and more peaceful. Outer order contributes to inner calm (a Zen thing), and when you don't feel well, calm and easy is good.

- ♥ Second: sticking to any resolution—no matter what it is—brings satisfaction. You've decided to make a change and you've stuck to it.

The payoff may not be immediately obvious, but with practice it will become second nature and you will reap the rewards. I've found that the easy consistency of making my bed each day was a great jumping-off point for making other small changes in the things I do have some control over (Mr. Duhigg's "Keystone Habit" idea). These small victories led me to feel better, a bit more capable, and happier. Less sick, less tired, a little sexier.

Being greeted by my lovely neat bedroom is its own reward each time I see it. It is my beautiful sanctuary, even though it's not fully enjoyed until bedtime.

> **"** *Success is the sum of small efforts, repeated day in and day out."*
>
> - Robert Collier

Since I have encouraged you to try making your bed each day, I had wondered how long it takes to create a new habit. I've always believed it was around 21 days, no more than three weeks.

Searching for an answer, I came across Gretchen Rubin's work again. She wrote another book, *Better Than Before: Mastering the Habits of Our Everyday Lives*, about how we make and break habits, and she wondered the same thing. According to her, a daily action takes an average of close to 66 days to become habit.

Two whole months. Well, Rome wasn't built in a day, was it?

A lot of variation is evident, both among people and habits. Some people are more "habit-resistant" than others, and some habits are harder to develop. Ms. Rubin said she found the study reassuring, and so do I, because it means that although everything won't be equally easy, with consistency and desire we can create new habits beneficial to our health and happiness.

Consider these two points from Gretchen Rubin's book:
1) By giving something up, you may gain.
2) What you do every day matters more than what you do once in a while.

> **❝** *Every accomplishment starts with the decision to try."*
>
> - Anonymous

I hope you'll try making your bed each day and see what happens. Here are my favorite tips on making your bed:

Simplify your bedding. Eliminate extra decorative pillows. Bedspread a pain? Use a duvet or comforter-cover over a feather duvet or hypo-allergenic synthetic. Duvet covers and shams are a simple, and affordable, way to update the look of your bedroom. You can change colors and fabrics according to the season. When the cover gets dirty, you just launder it, and put it back on your bed.

Sheets: Hate folding fitted bottom sheets? Why not use two flat sheets the way the hotels do? Much simpler.

Ready. Set. Go. Time yourself making your bed, just once. See how quick?

Spritz: Use a deliciously scented linen spray as you make your bed. One caveat: stick with all-natural products. You already have a chronic illness, why exacerbate it with indoor pollution?

Throw away sprays that are nothing more than chemical cover-ups *(such as Febreeze, AirWick, or Glade).*

Upgrade to a natural air spray like those made by Aura Cacia, Earth Friendly Products, or Zum. Those are a few I use.

KISS Tip: Make your own natural spritzer: Use a small 4 oz. spray bottle, 1.5 oz. distilled water, 1.5 oz. Vodka, and 15-20 drops of a clear natural essential oil of your choosing. I love Lavender in the bedroom to help me sleep, and lemon, grapefruit, or mint in the kitchen. Pick your favorites and make a combination that appeals just to you.

Spoil Yourself: As a finishing touch, add a small (or a large) vase of your favorite flowers to your bedside table or nightstand.

> " *I guarantee that developing new, positive habits will pay off. Pick a healthy habit or two you want to develop, and commit to give them a trial run for just two months. Once you're in the habit of bringing a nutritious lunch to work, or fitting in some meditation or yoga, and making your bed each morning, you won't even have to think about it anymore. Then the benefits of less stress, great food, and a sexier environment will be yours to enjoy.*"

FEED YOUR HEAD

In computer science, one concept states that the quality of the output is determined by the quality of the input. It is shortened to GIGO, which means "garbage in, garbage out."

It's the same with our mind and our body. The things we fill our time with, the foods we eat, the people we pay attention to, and especially the thoughts we consistently think, all become our reality. All of that is our "input."

If we want our reality to change, we have only to change our thoughts, because they control everything else we do. We must become aware of what we think, and we can do this by looking around ourselves. If what you see isn't exactly what you want, then it's time to set about changing it.

This could mean examining how we spend our spare time and what we fill our minds with.

- Do you spend your night watching reality TV so that you can escape your reality?

- Do you spend your spare time cruising social media for distraction, or as a way of feeling connected?

- Do you spend your time shopping online for things you don't really need?

- Do you read only romance novels or sci-fi fantasy, dreaming of rescue, or of escape to another world?

All of those activities are perfectly understandable. But if you keep doing what you've been doing, you'll keep getting what you've been getting. If you love what you have, that's great. If you don't, change where you focus your thoughts and your time.

Time isn't an unlimited resource, I'm sure you've realized you have only so many hours in a day, and only so many days on the planet.

Recognize that both you and your time are precious.

> 66 *All that we are is the result of what we think and have thought. What we are is founded on our thoughts, made up of our thoughts."*
>
> - Buddha

Social media wasn't the norm when I first became ill. Instead, I spent all day lying on the couch staring mindlessly at the food television networks. I fantasized about Ina Garten, "The Barefoot Contessa," inviting me for lunch and including me in her circle of friends. I felt lonely, and she was surrounded by good food and dear, smart friends.

Maybe one day I will meet her, but my point is, lying on the couch fantasizing was all I did, all day, for almost two months. I finally realized something needed to change. And that something was me, not my television.

Now, I often hear women complain that social media is taking up too much of their time, that they can't get anything done because of it. Remember - you're the boss.

Try this: take a limited social-media-semi-sabbatical for 40 days. Why forty? It's long enough to begin building a new habit, and yet short enough that you can consider undertaking it. And forty days is significant in Jewish, Christian, Islamic, and Hindu faiths, so it's a time period familiar to most of us. And really, what's forty days in the grand scheme of things?

My suggestion is this: check in on your social media three times a day, once in the morning, once in the afternoon, and once more after dinner or before bed. Give yourself 15-20 minutes each time. If you want to, you could announce you are doing it, and when you will check in. You can post it as your status. You can leave it as a recorded message on your phone. Resist the temptation to check-in when you are bored, or stuck, or feel sad or lonely.

But, what will you do instead? Seek out inspiration rather than distraction:

- Look at Oprah's Book Club or the *New York Times* bestseller list and take some time daily to read.
- Watch something new-to-you; a TED talk, Super Soul TV on Oprah, a special guest on Marie Forleo's website.
- Join a mailing list for daily or weekly inspiration.
- Get a #Truthbomb delivered to your phone on an app by Danielle LaPorte.
- Read nutritious cooking magazines that speak to your health/ wellness needs.
- Read a biography or an autobiography of someone who overcame an obstacle.
- Go for a walk in nature. If it's bad weather, go walk in the mall and look at the designs in the windows.
- Listen to music.
- Meditate, or learn to meditate. I love doing my meditation with mindfulness bells.
- At home in the evenings, watch something without all the drama and hype. Try comedies or inspiring documentaries.
- Play games with the kids, do their homework with them, talk to them, read to them.
- No kids? Play cards or a game and relax with your partner.
- No partner? Groom your pets, take them out to play. No pets, either?
- Meet friends to work out, have a glass of wine and a conversation, see a movie, go for tea.
- Too tired to go out? Take a bubble bath, read something that delights you, relax on your sofa.

At the end of forty days, you can go back to exactly what you were doing. If you still want to.

REMEMBER, "FOR THINGS TO CHANGE, FIRST I MUST CHANGE."

The biggest benefit I found in choosing inspiration rather than distraction was that I began to feel better. In my body, in my mind, and in my heart. My spirits lifted, my compassion for myself grew, and so did my belief in my ability to make positive, long-lasting changes in my life.

I now believed I could change my life for the better and the proof came one morning. For a couple of years I'd viewed the handful of the pills I took each morning as, "all of this damned medicine." I didn't like having to take it, and resentfully swallowed all fourteen pills at the appointed time.

On this particular day, as I lay the pills out on the shiny black countertop, they looked like stars out in space. Like a constellation, Orion's Belt, or the Big Dipper. It was a turning point, and in that instant I had a shift in how I viewed them. They became my "constellation of wellness."

I knew why I was taking all of them, but I hadn't really been grateful. Because of them, I could enjoy doing my work and having an income, being with friends and family, and pursuing my dreams and interests.

I began saying "thank you" each morning when I took the pills, and I focused on my wellness, rather than my illnesses.

All of the changes and positive input had begun to pay off.

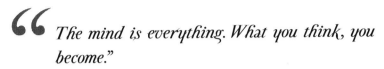 *The mind is everything. What you think, you become."*

— Buddha

I could share many, many more examples, but all of these new practices helped inspire me to get up off of the couch. They are the ones I continue to count on for inspiration.

What Inspires Me - A-Z

a. Listening to **A**braham-Hicks: regularly, for inspiration.

b. Moving my **B**ody: Nia classes, yoga, lifting weights, and walking. **B**aking, wheat-free - it's a challenge I love.

c. Julia **C**ameron: author *(The Artist's Way)* and Deepak **C**hopra: author, speaker, alternative medicine *(chopra.com)*

d. The **D**alai Lama: spiritual leader, author *(The Art of Happiness)* and Dr. Wayne **D**yer: author, speaker

e. The Fifth **E**lement: my favorite feel-good, futuristic, love story,

f. Marie **F**orleo: entrepreneur, author *(marieforleo.com)*

g. Elizabeth **G**ilbert: author, speaker *(Eat, Pray, Love)* and Seth **G**odin: author, entrepreneur, thought-leader

h. Louise **H**ay: author, publisher *(Heal Your Body)*

i. Pico **I**yer: author, essayist, and speaker (The Art of Stillness, The Open Road)

j. Time spent **J**ournaling each day, especially my gratitudes.

k. Robert **K**iyosaki: author and speaker *(Rich Dad, Poor Dad)*; Frida **K**ahlo: painter

l. Danielle **L**aPorte: author, speaker, thought-leader *(daniellelaporte.com)*

m. Tara **M**ohr: author, blogger (taramohr.com) **M**editation daily

n. Preparing **N**utritious food, beautifully. *(glutenfreegoddess.blogspot.com) (Pinterest)*

o. Watching anything on **O**prah: *(oprah.com)* Media, actress, philanthropist. Georgia **O**'Keeffe: The artist

p. Steven **P**ressfield: *(The Legend of Bagger Vance)* author. And **P**hotography

q. Taking some **Q**uiet time

r. Tony **R**obbins: Motivational speaker and author. **R**umi: A 13th century mystical poet

s. Linda **S**ivertsen: (BookMama.com) writer, teacher, author-whisperer

t. Watching **TED**talks: *(TED.com)* World's leading thinkers give an 18-minute talk.

u. This quote by **U**sher: "We all possess exactly what we need to be our greatest selves."

v. Richard Branson, and the **V**irgin Group: Entrepreneur, investor, author, philanthropist

w. Marianne **W**illiamson: *(A Return to Love)* author and speaker

x. Putting an **"x"** through something on my to-do list for the day

y. Taking **Y**oga classes, or doing guided Yoga nidra at home, and **Y**ouTube.com for videos

z. Rereading *Zen and the Art of Motorcycle Maintenance* by Robert Pirsig

YOU ARE WHAT YOU EAT

*First, a disclaimer: I am not a nutritionist; I don't even play one on TV. I've been cooking fresh, natural foods for 45 years. Preparing good food beautifully, and enjoying it, are two passions of mine. All of these ideas are my own, unless otherwise noted. Always check with your doctor before trying something new.

The group of preventable lifestyle diseases: hypertension, diabetes, obesity, and diseases related to smoking, and alcohol abuse, are all within our control. Which is, of course, why they are called preventable.

Unfortunately, I learned that eating well won't necessarily keep anyone from becoming ill. I ate exceptionally well, exercised regularly, and still developed a couple of chronic illnesses. But continuing to eat well and exercise has helped me manage these illnesses, and to feel as good as I do.

It's simple, really. You can't feel well if you don't feed your body well. And eating well depends upon your particular illness; it would be different for someone with diabetes than for someone with celiac disease. Eating nutritious foods that are right for me and drinking lots of water every day keep me feeling my best, with the added benefit of keeping me in great shape.

> **"** *One simple rule: If it came from a plant, eat it. If it was made in a plant, don't."*
>
> - Michael Pollan

*Note:** Foods are not healthy, or unhealthy. Healthy is the state of being in good health. People are healthy, or they're not. Foods are nutritious, or they're not. So, we should eat nutritious foods in order to become, and stay, healthy.

People always ask me, "What do you eat?" They're excited to know my secret, until I tell them what I eat. As it turns out, they don't want to not eat what I don't eat. And that's where I will start, with what I choose to avoid:

- ♥ Most packaged foods and mixes
- ♥ Conventional lunch meats and bacon which contain nitrites and nitrates,
- ♥ Frozen meals, packaged foods, canned vegetables or soups
- ♥ Fast food - McDonald's, Wendy's, KFC, Chick Fil-A, etc.
- ♥ Artificial sweeteners, colors, flavorings, or high-fructose corn syrup
- ♥ Inexpensive, color-added, artificially flavored yogurts
- ♥ Commercial beef, pork, and chicken containing hormones, steroids, antibiotics
- ♥ Most farm-raised fish
- ♥ Ice cream - I do better with an occasional non-dairy coconut milk treat
- ♥ Gluten-free replacement foods - often poor-quality ingredients
- ♥ Soda, sports drinks, vitamin waters
- ♥ Wheat *(and a few other grains, because they create symptoms for me)* which includes breads, pizza, cake, cookies

*Note:** There's a trend right now to avoid gluten and wheat. Wheat itself is not bad or evil, nor is gluten—which is a protein found in wheat, barley and rye—unless you have celiac disease, are gluten-sensitive, or are allergic to wheat. Going "gluten-free" only to replace all of the wheat products with poor quality substitutes won't make you lose weight or become any healthier.

It's odd, but out of my whole list, as soon as I say I don't eat bread, people's eyes glaze over and I feel an instantaneous disconnect. Some will simply say, "Oh." Case closed, end of conversation.

Some moan, "But I love bread. I could never do that!"

I smile and tell them I understand. Trust me, I do.

But some aren't satisfied and want to argue with me. "What about pasta? What about pizza? Are you kidding me? What about cookies? Cake, too? Croissants? Bagels? I could never do that!"

I ran into a woman I hadn't seen in years, and in our conversation she told me she was having inflammatory problems. I suggested she think about giving a Paleo or Primal diet a try for two weeks since it worked so well for my issues with an inflammatory disease process.

After arguing "at" me about not eating bread products for more than ten minutes, she finally said, "Forget it. I'd rather take muscle-relaxers, and go to the hospital periodically, than give up that much."

I was stunned. Yet I know many people who'd rather suffer and take drugs for their pain than alter their diets to see if they'd be pain-free. I don't understand the resistance.

I do, however, understand our love for baked goods. Fresh-baked bread has always been my idea of heaven, and, to add insult to injury, I'm a great baker. I learned to make fresh bread in the mid-1970s, and baked twice a week for years rather than buy the commercial white bread that was available. I found it relaxing to tend to it, then have the aroma of baking bread fill our home. I took pleasure in sending my son to school with a fresh sandwich in his lunch-box.

Once the person I'm speaking to accepts that I don't eat wheat, the next question usually is, "Well, then what DO you eat?" As if we live on wheat alone. But if you consume a standard American diet (whose initials are SAD) you pretty much do live on processed refined wheat alone.

Most pantries contain: bags and boxes of cookies, chips, crackers, pretzels, cereals, spaghetti, pasta, ramen noodles, toaster pastries, pancake mixes, cornbread and biscuit mixes, cake and cookie mixes, and canned and dehydrated packaged soups and gravies. Most manufactured food contains wheat.

An incredible variety of microwaveable frozen foods, all based around convenience, are very affordably priced because of their poor-quality and inexpensive ingredients.

They all contain wheat, too. And wheat, along with sugar and other inexpensive, poor-quality ingredients, comprises most commercial fast foods.

66 *You don't have to cook fancy or complicated masterpieces - just good food from fresh ingredients."*

- Julia Child

Make the switch back to nutritious foods. Phase them in, one or two at a time. Yes, it costs a little more because real ingredients cost more than manufactured ones. For an example, compare fresh-squeezed orange juice to a pitcher of orange flavored Kool-Aid. Big difference, right?

Good food isn't cheap and cheap food isn't good. It may be convenient, but it's not necessarily good for your health. And that's priceless, which I'm sure you realize. Give yourself a nutritional advantage. Your health is the best reason to eat well, and the second best reason is to set a good example for your children, if you have any.

Lecture over.

Note: If you're new to the idea of eating fresh natural foods, an anti-inflammatory food pyramid might be a good place to begin since most autoimmune disorders are a form of inflammation. Dr. Andrew Weil, a favorite on Oprah's show, and a favorite resource of mine, has one on his website. Dr. Terry Wahls has a protocol she used to get M.S. under control. You can find both online. You can also ask your doctor for a referral to a dietitian who specializes in autoimmune disorders, or to a functional medicine physician.

Let me share what I DO EAT:

- ♥ Lean grass-feed beef.
- ♥ Pork, bacon, and lunchmeats that are antibiotic-free, nitrate- and nitrite-free.
- ♥ Organic chicken and turkey
- ♥ Cage-free natural eggs
- ♥ Wild fish
- ♥ Fruits and berries, both fresh and frozen
- ♥ Vegetables, both fresh and frozen
- ♥ Nuts, natural nut butters (without added sugar), and seeds of all sorts
- ♥ Coconut milk and coconut water
- ♥ Dried fruits: raisins (especially golden raisins) dried cranberries, dates, dried plums, figs, and apricots
- ♥ Almond milk and hemp milk
- ♥ Small amounts of natural yogurt, organic cheese, heavy cream in my organic coffee
- ♥ Herb teas with honey. Maple syrup on occasional wheat-free pancakes.
- ♥ And heavenly smoothies, some 70% dark chocolate, and occasional home-made, wheat-free desserts,

Do I cheat? Sure, I occasionally cheat when we go out. I already admitted I'm not a saint. Sometimes the cheat is worth it, other times, for who-knows-what-reason, I pay a price for my indulgence. Which makes me more inclined to stay the course and find other things to bring me pleasure.

The best part of all of this, is that I RARELY FEEL DEPRIVED of anything. Except pizza. So far, I've been disappointed in most of the wheat-free pizzas. Oh, well. I find it hard to understand why people think giving up non-nutritious, fake food is going to deprive them of anything. Maybe a couple of dollars, their lack of energy, and some excess weight, but I can't imagine what else.

> ❝ *Don't eat anything your great-grandmother wouldn't recognize as food."*
>
> - Michael Pollan

A world full of beautiful, fresh, and nutritious food is already out there, and you have a choice to become healthier every single time you go to the grocery store. Shopping around the perimeter of the grocery store is where you will find all of the fresh foods: produce, meats, fish, dairy, and eggs. Use a list so you aren't tempted to buy what you don't need, and to be sure you do get the nutritious foods that will help you feel your best.

Shop at a time of day when you have the energy for it and don't feel rushed or pressured. Don't bring your children to the grocery store with you. Children want what they see on television, and it's all processed food. You don't need to argue or explain why you're buying what you're buying. If you can make arrangements for them, do so. Then everybody wins.

Start slowly, phase out one or two processed foods each week, and replace them with fresh, real food. Luncheon meats, hot dogs, and bacon are available without nitrates and nitrites. You can choose peanut butter and almond butter, even sunflower seed butter, that is only nuts and a dash of salt. Look for real fruit spreads. Real yogurt, hormone-free milk, applesauce that is unsweetened and delicious, and fruit cups in natural juice for their treats. Go to the store with an open mind and a sense of curiosity.

Learn to make a favorite, such as pizza, fresh at home using real ingredients. Natural crusts are available in the freezer aisle. Buy a natural sauce, (I'm a Newman's fan, love his flavors and philanthropy) and a variety of nutritious toppings, and have a family night dinner. Imagine your family all participating and bonding over an easy homemade meal. Serve a big salad and have a fruit plate for dessert. Skip the soft drinks, and offer a pitcher of colorful herb tea, or water with lemons and limes in it.

As Julia Child would say, *"Bon Appetit!"*

WATCH YOUR LANGUAGE

We are at a point in our evolution where we need to choose our words more carefully because, unfortunately, we have become unconscious of what we say. In our collective efforts to rid ourselves of what we don't want, we have waged a war against everything: drugs, poverty, women, obesity, crime, and terror. We fight heart disease, illiteracy, colds, and mental illness. We battle cancer. We fight for reform and for human rights. We fight for peace.

We go out into the world prepared to do battle daily. How exhausting.

As we have conversations with friends, associates, and even strangers, we casually toss out that we hate most everything. "Don't you just hate that?"

"Yeah, I hate it when that happens!"

We'll use "lethal" words about something we covet: "That dress is to die for."

And with the same ease, we say we'd kill for something else, "Damn, I'd kill for a cookie!"

All of this parlance has become a part of the way we communicate. I just read a two-page magazine article entitled, "5 Reasons Your Back is Killing You," by Nancy Szokan. Let's face it, if the article had offered five reasons why your back hurts so much, it wouldn't have had the same impact.

The point I'm making is, with so much negativity built into our everyday language, we don't even notice it anymore. Consequently, we put this negativity "out there" into the world millions of times a day.

Here's why this is important: our words have power, and our thoughts create. Since this is the case, it only makes sense we should pay more attention to both.

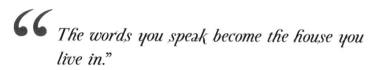

“ *The words you speak become the house you live in."*

— Hafiz

Language, or choice of words, affects those of us with chronic illnesses. When we live with illnesses, we tend to claim them as our own. In conversation we say, "my arthritis," "my ulcers," and even "my cancer."

Not much wiggle-room there, is there? I've found that by not owning sickness we leave ourselves room for healing. I'm not saying to deny you are dealing with an illness, but I am saying, don't own it. Okay, you're game, but how can you say it differently?

First, stop calling it "mine." It's not really anything you want, or would have chosen, like a cute pet, or a new car, or your friends, is it? I knew a woman who lived with cancer for a long time, and she always called it "my cancer." Another woman I know calls her ulcerative colitis, "my constant companion."

So, first thing we will do is quit saying, "my_____." When I talk about it, I use the term "having" an illness, one day I may not have it anymore. Or I call it, "the autoimmune disorder, or the bone-marrow disease."

Here's another: I'm sure you've asked someone how they're doing only to have them respond along the lines of, "Lousy, my allergies are killing me!" Double-whammy, my allergies are killing me. We could simply say we're having trouble with allergies today.

Often, we'll say, "I'm sick," or "I am so exhausted." I am is another way of owning something, by claiming it or labeling it.

It would be better for us to replace "I'm _____" with "I feel _____." It took me a while to stop saying, (whining, actually) "I'm so exhausted." I caught myself over and over, then I'd correct myself and change it to "I feel so exhausted today."

In making that one conscious change, I've gone from labeling myself, to simply stating how I feel.

On Oprah's show, Joel Osteen said, "Whatever you say after you say 'I Am' is going to come looking for you."

Wow, what a thought! What do we want to have come looking for us? Let's move toward our healing by watching our language and becoming aware of which words we choose to use.

Since our words can shape our future, let's make it a healthy and fulfilling one.

> **"** *Since everything is a reflection of our minds,*
> *everything can be changed by our minds."*
>
> - Buddha

Postscript: I just received a letter from M.D. Anderson Cancer Center in Houston. They have crossed through the word "cancer" on all of their stationery. It now reads: MD Anderson Center, Making Cancer History.

Lovely affirmation, isn't it?

THERE'S NO RUT IN ROUTINE

Routines are something I thought I didn't like. I feared they would make me feel less free-spirited, less able to do things on a whim. I was always afraid of being an automaton, stuck in a rut. Aside from keeping consistent hours at work, I told myself I preferred to hang-loose.

But I regularly exercised four times a week. And my laundry and grocery shopping always got done on Monday. But other than those things, I didn't want to get committed to a routine.

I liked the freedom to spontaneously grab dinner with friends, or to skip dinner altogether and munch popcorn as I read in the bathtub. I wanted to be able to catch a late movie, or stay up all night reading. I traveled when I wanted, with very little planning. I enjoyed exotic foods and drinks with my friends. I slept late on Sundays.

Two things in life can bring that type of lifestyle to an end: Having children. Or becoming ill.

Just one of them pulled the reins up short for me. I can't imagine having to manage both. Well, actually, I can imagine it, and I see how difficult it would be. I've talked to many women who struggle with both, and I am firmly convinced the best way to take care of yourself (first, or course) in order to take care of your others, is to establish a good routine.

THIS IS A FIRST

I never thought I'd be one to embrace a routine, and I certainly never thought I'd suggest one to anybody else. But now I realize that routines aren't ruts. An old joke goes, "What's the difference between a rut and a grave? Six feet."

Without my routines I might already be in my grave. Let me show you how establishing routines worked for me, and offer you ideas on why you'd want to establish them for yourself. And, yes, I'm going all Aretha Franklin here by spelling it out.

"R" - doing things REGULARLY.

1) Take your medicines regularly, in the prescribed amounts, and on schedule.

2) Eat at regular hours. Don't skip meals. Plan ahead, sit down, and eat something nutritious.

3) Go to bed and rise at approximately the same time each day. This helps keep all of your other schedules on track. Of course, luxuriate on your day off, by sleeping in if you can.

4) Exercise regularly. Anything from walking to lifting weights, or a gentle yoga class. Just moving helps us stay or become strong, both physically and emotionally. It decreases stress. If ever you needed to exercise, now is the time.

5) Rest. Set aside 15 minutes a day to just sit quietly or lie down. If you have children, include them in this quiet time by explaining you all need it to recharge. You can teach them a valuable lesson about your worth by demonstrating good self-care. You'll also create bonding time.

"O" - is for ORGANIZED

1) Make a list, check it twice. Get a chalkboard, white board, or corkboard, and use it. We can't remember everything when we're ill, and sometimes important

things slip through the cracks. I also love sticky notes, but you know how that goes. I have the little buggers everywhere. Not very sexy. A board is great place to put your med schedule, doctor's appointments and numbers, and the pharmacy number.

2) Keep a grocery list stuck to your board or the fridge. Make one on the computer, print off a few copies, and stick them up there. As you use things up, check the box. Next time you make a run to the store, or someone does it for you, you have a list.

3) Your board is also a great place to list things you want to ask your doctor on your next visit. With so many different doctors, we need to relay information as well as ask questions. Lists, baby!

4) If you tend to be disorganized (closets are crammed full, laundry basket always overflowing), think about putting things in order. Chaos is not conducive to healing. Nor is it very sexy.

5) Drinking enough water is a challenge for many of us. Get organized here by buying a BPA-free bottle or pitcher and filling it daily. As a treat, add a few berries, mint leaves, or lemon and lime. Then drink it. You'll never have to wonder whether you drank enough, and you won't suffer from dehydration.

"U" - look for the UPSIDE

1) Ludicrous, I know. You've got a chronic illness and I'm suggesting you look for an upside. But if you look, you will find one. A "glass is half-full" attitude is the way to go, since a positive attitude has been proven to be good for your mental and emotional outlook, and thus, your overall health.

2) Stay present with just what is. You're here now. Don't deny it, minimize it, or "awful-ize" it.

3) Remember: new medicines, new treatments, new discoveries happen every day. In the meantime, we need to take the best possible care of ourselves so we will be here for them.

4) When I was diagnosed with E.T., I realized I might not have the whole life I had envisioned ahead of me. This awareness gave me some clarity. I learned what was really important to me, and quit putting things off. I tried new things and worried less about failing.

5) And the best upside of all: I found out I am a much stronger woman than I ever thought I could be. You are, too!

"T" - make TIME for your needs

1) Set aside some "Me Time" each day. Make it non-negotiable. Declare it. You can lie down and put your feet up. You can meditate. You can take a bath. You can listen to music, or you can make a cup of tea and simply stare out a window. Make this YOUR time to recharge.

2) Make time for movement: a stroll around the block with your phone turned off, a beginner's yoga class, or a barre class, or kettle-bells or free-weights, if you are up to it. Again, make your movement time sacrosanct.

3) Make time to meet with friends regularly. Outdoors, if possible. This way you have the benefit of friends and of fresh air. If you can be around water, even better. The negative ions bodies of water give off are very, very good for us.

4) Make time for maintenance. A therapeutic massage, a Reiki session, a facial, a spray tan, a great pedicure and/or manicure. Visit your chiropractor, or your acupuncturist.

"I" - INVEST in yourself

1) Just because you have an illness doesn't mean your ideas and dreams must end. If anything, illness should galvanize things for you. If you've always wanted to paint, write, take language classes, learn to play piano, or dance, do it. If you need permission for something "so frivolous," I give you permission, and blessings.

2) Not loving your job? Begin to look for a different one better suited to you. Need more education to get where you want to be or to change fields? Do it. You only have one life to live, and it's up to you to choose how you will live it. Sometimes just this awareness alone brings all sorts of unexpected opportunities into your life.

3) Invest in your appearance. Get a good haircut that makes your life easy. If you color your hair, add that to your calendar and prioritize yourself. There's no point in coloring if you are consistently letting 3" of roots show. You aren't fooling anyone, and you'll feel bad each time you look in the mirror. Think about going natural. Talk to your stylist. Looking pulled-together is good for your mental health, and that's good for your physical health.

"N" - Remember, NOW is the only time there is

1) Stay present. It does no good to live in the past, in the time before you became ill. Grieving is normal. But after that, focus on today, focus on living.

2) Do the best you can each day, knowing it's normal to have both good, and not-as-good, days. We are always a work-in-progress. Work with what's there for you today and be gentle with yourself.

3) Now is the time to learn to ask for what you need or want. Don't hope someone will read your mind and give it to you. Ask for it, whatever "it" is.

4) Thinking about making some changes? Start today, because all you have is right now. Dream big. See your dreams as already accomplished. Then think about how great you are going to feel.

"E" - Create and conserve ENERGY

1) I risk sounding like a broken record, but both rest and exercise are vital. Exercise will give you more energy. If you're not well enough to exercise, go for a stroll.

2) Sometimes resting doesn't make me feel any better at all, but listening to a guided meditation, inspiring podcast, or watching a short video energizes me.

3) Take the kids to the park. Bring a picnic of nutritious snacks and watch them play. No kids? Take your dog. No dog? Take a book and spend some time reading. Watch clouds. Feel yourself relax.

4) Learn your limits. Once you know them, honor them. Learn when you can say "yes," and when to say "no." Even if it's your children or your partner. They will only respect your limits if you do, and martyrdom serves nobody.

5) Know the signs you're doing too much before you become overwhelmed. Energy is precious and can be mood-altering. Sometimes I feel like the Energizer Bunny, other times I feel as if I've been unplugged. Stay in touch with how you are feeling.

Rather than look at routines as hard-and-fast rules, I choose to see them as "my practice," a method to increase my overall health and well-being. I continue following them and improving on them, in order to support my healing and my sanity.

Merriam-Webster Dictionary defines PRACTICE as: "to do something again and again in order to become better at it, and to do (something) regularly or constantly as an ordinary part of your life."

I must admit, as much as I thought I disliked routines, it turns out I don't. Now I don't like getting too far out of my routines because I love the way my life is working, and I love the way I feel. Who knew?

PART TWO

Staying There

SECTION 1

What Is Sexy, After All?

First Thoughts

Everything has lead up to this chapter. Acceptance. Being here now. Recognizing the need for change in our lives. Developing gratitude for all we have. Speaking in a more life-affirming way. And caring for ourselves first, in order to take care of others.

By seeking sources of inspiration, we gather momentum and recharge our "batteries." Eating to support ourselves and creating routines will sustain us. All of this is intended to give us back our energy, confidence, and our joie de vivre.

When I've told people what I was writing about, most women were really excited, and most also knew someone they wanted an extra copy for. On the flip side, some women have defensively pointed out that being sexy isn't important to them, and never has been. I've had women ask why they should care about being sexy. Still others tell me wistfully that being sexy isn't on their radar since they don't even have the energy to think about it. To say that I understand is an understatement.

When talking about feeling sexy, women usually mean whether or not we feel like having sex. Or else we compare ourselves to the current trend of overt sexuality that is everywhere these days. How on earth can a real woman relate to that? Who, even with good health, can take care of a home, work, shop, cook, run-errands, and raise kids dressed in stilettos with her hair done, full make-up on, and everything pushed up and out?

To think about being sexy in only these terms is ludicrous, and taken in that context, I understand the question, and even the defensiveness. Our sexuality and our femininity are an integral and vibrant part of who we are as female human beings; it's the juicy part of our lives as women. Like a snowflake, it's individual and unique to each of us.

Without juiciness, engagement, and intimacy we can become uptight, withdrawn, and apathetic. We can give up on our appearance and our dreams. Both aging and illness could be considered valid reasons for not caring about being sexy anymore, but they can also be an excuse.

Giving up is a decision. It may be an unconscious decision, but we choose it. The good news is, you can also choose to get those lovin' feelings back. Here's what I really want you to know: sexy is not necessarily high heels, flowing hair, and cleavage. But it certainly can be. If you've decided that you can't live up to the image you have in your head, read on.

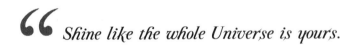

66 *Shine like the whole Universe is yours.*

- Rumi

MOVING BEYOND IMAGE

I did a couple of informal polls among my readers and friends. The first time I asked only women, "What makes you feel sexy?" and "What do you think is sexy?" Their responses were:

- ♥ Confidence. Strength. Passion. Intelligence.
- ♥ The ability to look someone in the eye.
- ♥ Fitness. Fearlessness. Attitude.
- ♥ Dressing-up. Sense of humor.
- ♥ Feeling pampered. Feeling pulled-together.

- ♥ Chemistry. Being comfortable in your skin.
- ♥ Dressing well. Beautiful lingerie. Genuineness. Self-love.
- ♥ Red lipstick.
- ♥ Loving life.
- ♥ A beautiful smile.

Then I did another informal poll on Facebook and invited both my male and female friends to respond. "What qualities do you consider sexy in a woman?" The responses were:

> Whimsy, self-confidence, great eyes and eye-makeup, confidence, caring and sensibility, compassion, kindness, sense of humor, smart, funny, humility, comfortable in her body, intelligence, kindness, mindfulness, intent, style, sensuality, great imagination, good figure, vibrant, fun personality.

Then, for good measure, I posed one last question only to women, "Describe sexuality or sexual energy in a sentence."

> "Sexual energy makes us feel vital."
>
> "Passionate and fierce – like a lioness."
>
> "It is tender, vulnerable, and intuitive."
>
> "Sexuality is vibrant and engaging."
>
> "Sexual energy is radiant."
>
> "Sexuality is about loving whatever body you're in, and enjoying it."
>
> "It's a comfort level with yourself that shows up as confidence."
>
> "It is more than just your willingness to have sex."
>
> "Sexiness keeps us engaged and connected."

I found it interesting is that the men's answers were a lot less sexually-oriented than I thought they'd be. While men all admitted that a "nice figure" or "great boobs" were a point of attraction, they said confidence, a sense of humor, being smart, and having a great personality were more important to the success of the relationship in the long run.

> " *In my opinion, sexiness comes down to three things: chemistry, sense of humor, and treatment of wait staff at restaurants."*
>
> - Rhoda Janzen

I found the most delightful post, "What Makes Someone Sexy?" by Leanne Shirtliffe in her blog, ironic.com.

In it, she tells a story about playing basketball in her driveway competing against her seven-year-old twins. She was feeling out of shape, and not very desirable. Her husband came home, and after watching her play for a while, he told her, "This is when I find you sexiest."

Naturally, she was confused because she was sweaty, out of breath, and not wearing any makeup. When she resisted the compliment, he explained what he found attractive was that she was unguarded, in her own world, and focused.

As a result, she started thinking about what made moms sexy. Her conclusion on what makes any adult sexy: "Confidence. Expertise. Passion. Humor. And clothes-that-fit-whatever-shape-or-size-you-are-right-now."

WHY SHOULD I CARE ABOUT BEING SEXY?

I'm going to answer that question with another question, "Why would you want to put the sexy part of yourself on the back-burner just because of a chronic illness?" We feel sexiest when we feel good about ourselves, when we like our lives, and feel well and full of energy. All of this can, of course, be challenging when we have a chronic illness.

If we're in a relationship, or want to be, we would do well to take good care of ourselves and nurture all parts of our sexuality. It's probably not a good idea to abandon this part of yourself if any romantic relationship is to endure. I've learned we must strive for balance, and we can't let everyday demands make us put our relationship last or take it for granted. Many relationships fall apart because of the pressure that living with chronic illness can place on them. While the divorce rate has declined in America, it tends to be higher among couples dealing chronic illness.

I had to rely on my partner to be my caregiver for a short while, but as soon as possible, I made myself do things again. I made an effort to look better than the zombie I still felt like. I went to my doctor's appointments alone, armed with my list of questions, and wrote down the answers one-by-one. I did the grocery shopping alone, took care of my own laundry, and I began cooking us dinners again and trying new Paleo recipes we'd both enjoy.

And I did this as much for myself, as for my fiancé. I wanted to regain my autonomy, and by extension, my confidence and sense of myself as a capable woman. I was worried about the effect that having my lover become my caretaker might create. I may have been overly sensitive about this, but I wanted to do my best to keep him as my sweetheart, and not have him feel that he was my nursemaid or my roommate.

I want to keep the romance alive as long as possible. Although I'm no youngster, and come to think of it, neither is he, my sensual side isn't something I was ready, or willing, to give up, even though I hadn't seen hide-nor-hair of it for months! As I began to feel better and started going for walks, my energy returned. And along with energy, the pleasure and comfort of "being back in my skin," rather than disconnected from my body, grew.

While our relationship benefited from all of these choices in the long run, I'm the one who really benefited every time I caught a glimpse of myself in the mirror. I remember seeing myself one day and thinking, "Hmmmnnn, I don't look nearly as bad as I feel!"

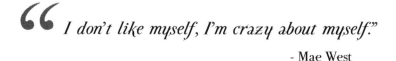 *I don't like myself, I'm crazy about myself."*

- Mae West

To be crazy about yourself, you have to take great care of yourself and choose to keep your "batteries" recharged. Even if you're single, you still want to feel engaged and interested in what's going on around you. A dear friend and her husband inspire me with their Date Night every week - they always go to the same chic restaurant and sit at "their corner" of the large modern bar. From here they can see all of the activity, visit with the owner, and watch the show in the kitchen. All while enjoying a cocktail, having dinner, and being sweethearts on a date.

Other things that are good for keeping you feeling desirable are:
- ♥ going out with dear friends
- ♥ a great massage
- ♥ an exercise class
- ♥ a manicure or pedicure in a quiet place
- ♥ meditating or sitting quietly for 15 minutes
- ♥ taking time to read a great book, maybe even something racy or romantic
- ♥ getting a fresh haircut or color
- ♥ clothing in sensual fabrics
- ♥ buying new lingerie
- ♥ a home environment conducive to the sexy side of ourselves: neat and tidy, a scented candle, a small vase of flowers
- ♥ date night - good for recharging your connection to each other

(Off-limits: discussing the kids, the pets, or household problems)

SURROUNDED BY SEXY

I like having the bathroom to myself to shower and get ready. I think it's sexier to have a bit of mystery about what goes on behind the scenes. To keep that mystery, I don't fill the shower with every face wash, douche, razor, loofah, scrub, shampoo, conditioner, body moisturizer, or self-tanner I use. I don't find clutter sexy, so I have everything easily accessible in baskets under my counter. I use it and put it back, maintaining a serene vibe.

I want all of the paraphernalia of illness to be out of sight too. I don't leave my medicines, hormone creams, or the blood-pressure cuff lying around just because I'll need them again later. (I realize it may not always be possible to put things away, depending on your illness, but if you can, find a way to organize the things you must have readily available.)

My neatness is about focusing on the vibration I want to live in. There is a method to my madness, of course. First, it's good Feng Shui for our living environment to be neat and orderly, allowing for maximum positive energy flow.

Second, it's the law of attraction: what you focus on, you get more of. I choose to focus on feeling happy, healthy, and beautiful by creating a space that reflects what I feel is beautiful. I want what I find sexy to be what's on display - a favorite bottle of perfume, a pair of earrings with sentimental value, a cherished piece of artwork, a few flowers.

Allow your personality, sense of style, and sensual side to shine through. Trust that you are always desirable. Focus on things you love. You will feel sexier if everywhere you look you see the beauty you've created, I promise.

" *I never said it would be easy, I only said it would be worth it.*"

- Mae West

THE PLEASURE PRINCIPLE

Consider the word pleasure for a minute. Where did you go with that? Most people think pleasure means sex, but in reality, sex means sex. From the root word plaisir, to please, the word pleasure means happy satisfaction, or enjoyment. People generally don't place enough emphasis on their pleasure. On hard work, sacrifice, and attainment, yes. On pleasure, not so much.

Pleasure (and there are so many kinds available) isn't usually very high on our priority list, both when we are well, and especially when we don't feel well, even though it has so many health benefits for us:

- ♥ Pleasure tells blood vessels to widen and relax, which lowers our blood pressure
- ♥ Pleasure releases dopamine, providing us with feelings of enjoyment and reinforcing our motivation
- ♥ Pleasure releases nitric oxide, playing a role in reducing inflammation
- ♥ Pleasure releases beta-endorphins which decrease pain and create euphoria
- ♥ Pleasure releases vasopressin, which increases feelings of bonding
- ♥ Pleasure releases oxytocin which increases feelings of bonding and trust

Think about the last time you had a night out with friends, laughing and having fun. Remember how relaxed you were, and the camaraderie you felt in that situation.

Here's another: think about sex and orgasm. Now recall the sense of well-being and connectedness you feel afterward, that desire to cuddle, feeling safe and secure.

Pleasure and the host of chemicals it releases into your body brought you all of those feelings. Now tell me - why wouldn't we want to feel pleasure more often? Oh, that's right, you don't feel well, everything hurts, and, on top of all of that, you're too tired to think about pleasure.

I recently learned about Regena Thomashauer, the leader of the Pleasure Revolution. Her avid fans call her Mama Gena, and I saw why when I watched her on an inspiring TED Talk where she said most of us view pleasure as "a seedy street in a bad neighborhood that we don't want to go down, and that we don't want anyone else to go down either!"

For Mama Gena, pleasure is anything BUT a seedy street. Pleasure is what lights us up and ignites us, and she believes it is the "secret elixir," the vital nutrient missing from most of our lives. We are just starting to realize all of pleasure's benefits to our health, mental-health, and wellness.

I know I am repeating myself, but we haven't been taught to take care of ourselves FIRST, or maybe even at all. On the contrary, we've been taught to take care of everyone else first, and as Mama Gena says, "Whatever crumbs are left over, those are yours!"

> ❝ *To keep the body in good health is a duty, otherwise we shall not be able to keep our mind strong and clear.*"
>
> - Buddha

We have been raised to believe that this is how a good wife/mother/daughter should act, but let's face it, if you look throughout history, martyrdom never ended well. When you don't take care of yourself, putting yourself way down the list instead, you feel bad and everybody loses. When you take care of yourself first, allowing yourself to feel increased pleasure and less stress, you're more available and have more to give. Everybody wins!

As women, we are hardwired for pleasure, and a lack of it results in stress hormones coursing through our bodies, producing irritation and stress-induced illnesses. One thing is certain: a lack of self-care can be self-destructive. Mama Gena said, "Where we are right now with pleasure is where we were forty years ago with fitness!" We all understand the need for exercise, and the benefits of fitness. We also know that getting there involves effort, right? Here's the biggest boon to pleasure - no work, all play!

Dr. Christiane Northrup also believes we need pleasure in order to be happy and healthy, and increased nitric oxide is the key. "Most of us don't produce enough of it to keep us vibrantly healthy."

Nitric oxide is a gas made naturally by the body which expands blood vessels, allowing more oxygen to reach our heart, brains, and other important organs. Without enough, we can feel fatigued and worn out, and often turn to sugar and alcohol to give ourselves that boost we are craving.

How do we get more of this feel-good chemical in our body? It's easy to boost nitric oxide naturally, and here's what we need:

- ♥ A balanced and healthy diet. Include dark chocolate, watermelon, pomegranate, cranberries, oranges, peanut butter, walnuts, pistachios, brown rice, spinach, beets, garlic, kale, onion, black tea, cayenne pepper, honey, salmon, and shrimp.

- ♥ Exercise, because when your heart pumps harder more nitric oxide is released.

- ♥ Meditation or quiet time - as little as 15 minutes a day. (this can be done in 5-minute sessions of that's even easier)

- ♥ Thinking joyful thoughts - all it takes is 17 seconds of focused thought.

- ♥ Laughter - Read or watch something that makes you laugh. Do something silly.

- ♥ Touching, and being touched by others, is an essential need we never outgrow.

♥ Get a good massage as often and as regularly as you can schedule it in.

♥ Regular sex is important (no, not as opposed to the kinky kind). Foster your sexuality; from simply holding hands, to cuddling and caressing, sex releases oxytocin and endorphins, the same as exercise does.

♥ Self-love: masturbation also has health benefits. It reduces stress, helps offset insomnia, boosts metabolism, and stimulates the production of endorphins to ease your pain and stress. Just in case you need to hear this: Guilt is optional.

Bottom line, the more pleasure you can pack into your life on a daily basis, the less sick and tired you are likely to feel. Maybe you'll even start feeling sexy again!

THE KISS PRINCIPLE

I don't remember the first time I heard about KISS – short for the (rude) directive to "keep it simple, stupid." Must have been in high school.

Over the years I have always reminded myself to "keep it simple," when I was becoming overwhelmed, or stressing-out about something I needed to do. However—and this is really important—I changed the "stupid" part in order to speak more kindly to myself. Remember, our words have power. When I did this, it became "keep it simple, sweetie." A much nicer way to talk to yourself, if you're going to talk to yourself at all, don't you think?

When I felt better after having been so sick and tired, the saying evolved one last time as I started making changes to take better care of myself. Now it's "keep it simple, sexy."

Any time I wonder what choice to make, or what would be the best solution for a clothing or design dilemma, I think KISS and choose the sexiest option available to me.

This dress or that one? Which will make me feel sexier every time I wear it? This color for the bath re-do, or that? Well, which would look sexier in the bath? What to make for dinner tonight? What's simple and nutritious, yet still elegant? Can I find a pair of shoes that are both comfortable and sexy? Thanks, I'll take two pair! Making choices becomes easy when you narrow down the options, and I've narrowed them down to just one: do I find this simple-and-sexy, or not?

ARRIVING AT KISS

A few years ago, I traveled to the Texas coast for a long weekend with my sweetheart. The second day we were there the weather turned rainy and cool, and during breakfast we wondered what to do with the day. We were on the motorcycle and had planned on riding and stopping somewhere for lunch, but the weather wasn't going to cooperate for a while. We decided to walk along the beach and gather seashells. As we left the hotel, we each grabbed a Styrofoam cup from the coffee bar to hold our shells.

Walking along the water's edge, talking and scouting for treasure, I became overwhelmed by all of the options. I know it sounds silly, but I didn't want a lot of shells, just a few. Just the right ones. Should we pick up the white shells or the black ones? What about the rusty looking ones, they were pretty, too. Did we want them with holes in them or not? Did we want the scalloped ones, or spiral ones?

Finally, we decided to pick up only the small, black, scalloped shells because right after chrome, black is our favorite color. We found lovely obsidian-colored shells no bigger than a dime mixed in with all of the other shells, and after an hour, the sun came out, the clouds cleared and we had all the shells we needed. The shells sit in a small snifter on my windowsill, and they are a reminder of the valuable lesson I learned that day: narrowing down my choices was much more freeing than dealing with too many choices. It allowed me to focus and to have fun, by keeping it simple.

Barry Schwartz, a psychologist and the author of *The Paradox of Choice: Why More is Less*, confirmed what I learned when gathering seashells - that having too many options can in fact lead to paralysis. He went into delightful detail in a TED talk, and the take-away is this: more choice does not equal more freedom.

With all of the choices available to us, for everything we DO choose, we don't get to choose anything else. He called these "opportunity costs," and these costs can lead to regret, second-guessing ourselves over the decision we've made, and dissatisfaction with our choice because it didn't live up to our expectations.

We are flooded daily with stimuli: on our TVs, computers, cell phones, tablets, and magazines. Advertising, everywhere we look. All of this increases our stress in subtle ways, which in turn can elevate our blood pressure and create insomnia and anxiety, along with neck and shoulder pain. Excess stimulation can also create constant tiredness and a feeling of being overwhelmed, one of the last things I need.

With everything else I am required to make decisions about daily, I don't have the energy left to get stressed out over another choice, so I defer to my KISS guideline: Will this choice make my life easier? Where is the sexiness in this? It all comes down to those two things: is it simple and is it sexy? Make this your mantra.

> " *Although I'm not one for austerity, I think there is something to simplicity – the mental, logistical and physical spareness that brings a few key priorities into focus."*
>
> - Mark Sisson

While I'm not one for austerity either, I do believe in making life as simple as possible. The less we have going on around us demanding to be addressed, the more we can pay attention to a few important priorities, namely our physical health, our spirit, and having more energy to enjoy ourselves and our loved ones.

One way I work toward simplicity is by playing a game with myself: if I buy or bring something new into the house, I must find one or two things to give away. I am working toward the minimalist lifestyle I'd like to be living. More stuff equals more to take care of, and I don't want to spend the energy I do have taking care of a house full of stuff anymore.

Leo Babuta wrote a beautiful article entitled, "72 Ideas to Simplify Your Life." In it he pointed out that living a simple life has a different meaning to everybody. And getting to a point of simplicity isn't always simple. He said it's a journey, not a destination, and it can often be two steps forward, and one backward.

Who among us doesn't know that dance? I focus on the fact that even when I have moved one step backward, I am still one step farther along than I was. We're always one step ahead when we're trying.

He offered lots of ideas for simplifying our life, but he stated that there are really only two steps:

1. Identify what's important
2. Eliminate everything else

Simple, isn't it? Take a few minutes, perhaps over a cup of tea, and figure out what is really important to you. Here is what I found for myself when I did this:

♥ **I want to live simply yet beautifully.**

♥ **I am open to growth and learning in order to become healthier.**

♥ **I want to share my experiences using creativity and my sense of humor.**

Before I could get to the "living simply yet beautifully" part, I had to get rid of a lot of stuff. I owned clothes I never wore but kept anyway because, well, you know. I had multiples of household appliances since we had merged two households. And overall, there was just too much to take care of.

Here's what I learned: go for quality, not quantity. I decided to have fewer things, but have them be things I love, that are well made, and which will add value to my life.

Ask yourself this: Are your closets bulging at the seams? Basement full? Keeping your cars in your driveway because all of your extra stuff is in the garage? Are you paying for a storage unit full of things you never even see?

These things all sap our energy, and every time I opened a closet door or walked out into the garage, I could feel my own energy spiral down, down, down. The emotional weight of all that stuff was a tremendous burden.

After a challenging downsize and move, from 3400 sq.ft. to 1100 sq.ft., I needed help narrowing down my remaining possessions to only ones that I loved. Friends raved about a book by Marie Kondo called *The Life-Changing Magic of Tidying Up*, which was a *New York Times* bestseller. I bought it and read it cover-to-cover.

What I like best about her method is that, although it's more detail-oriented than I could ever imagine being, IT WORKS. It was actually fun. She's got a million rules, but they are mercifully simple:

- ♥ Tidy by category: For example, do all of your cosmetics and toiletries at the same time. Do all of your books and magazines at once. Do all of your clothes at once. She shows why doing a room at a time doesn't work.
- ♥ How do you know what to keep? Only keep things that spark joy for you.
- ♥ Once sorted, discard everything you're not keeping, right then, intensely and completely.
- ♥ When you put what you're keeping back in your dresser, never pile things. She has her own unique folding method, and it works beautifully.
- ♥ Her last rule, and she is adamant on this point: don't change the rules to suit yourself.

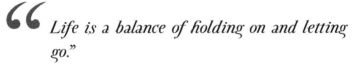

" Life is a balance of holding on and letting go."

- Rumi

After I organized my closet and dresser, I met a friend for coffee to compare notes on how our tidying was going. We both had a good laugh about trying to fold thong underwear using her method, some things just need to be stacked. Sometimes you've got to break the rules to suit yourself.

By keeping only what gives you joy, showing respect and honor to all that you have, and putting your house in order, Marie Kondo believes your whole life can benefit. And, I agree. I believe we can bring ourselves closer to wholeness/wellness. Less visual clutter equals less stress, and less stress equals a healthier sexier you.

The more I gave away items that were no longer useful or which had been a burden or obligation to maintain, the lighter and calmer I felt. Lighter and calmer definitely feels sexier. It's all right if there are empty spaces, allow those spaces to become filled with appreciation and healing.

Now, as Leo Babuta says, "Make a list of your favorite simple pleasures, and sprinkle them throughout your day." Buy yourself a bunch of flowers when you go to the grocers, or a couple of bottles of sparkling water. Buy some incense or a scented candle. Pick up a piece of dark chocolate.

Treat yourself to something wonderful. You deserve it.

ASK FOR HELP

Still can't get beautifully organized? Having trouble simplifying? Hire a professional. Whatever you don't want to do, or don't enjoy - there is someone who loves to do it, and is good at it. That's what makes the world go around! If hiring someone isn't the answer for you, recognize that your friends and loved ones want to help you, but need to know what they can do. Ask if they'd be willing to share their natural talents.

- ♥ Have a friend who is amazingly organized? Ask her help to bring order to your place and then make a run to a local charity to donate your excess. Many people need what you don't.
- ♥ Books and magazines piled everywhere, but you can't bear to part with them? Again, get a friend to help. By letting go of the ones you really don't love, you can focus on the ones you do. And you may even reread a few! There are hospitals and nursing homes that would love your excess books. Get them to those who really need them.
- ♥ Medical bills too much to deal with? Find a friend or professional who can get a handle on everything for you.

I had a dear friend who was overwhelmed by her medical bills, student loan papers, and the forms the insurance company sent after every doctor visit. Since she was so sick, they piled up. And piled up. These are one of the few things that can't be ignored. Get a champion to help you out.

When everything is simplified and in order, YOU will feel more in-control and on top of things. During a relapse or flare, it will make life easier if everything is in its place. You can focus solely on resting and getting back to beautiful.

KISS AND GET DRESSED

Let's talk about clothes. Let's talk about the idea that getting your clothes organized will make you feel more comfortable and more confident. Which will in turn raise your energy and make you feel better.

Marie Kondo's rule is: keep only what sparks joy. Any article of clothing that truly sparks joy would by nature be one that makes you both feel good, and look good. Rarely have I seen a woman look bad in something she loves!

But first, let's start with the "sick and tired" default outfit: yoga clothes, sweatpants, and hoodies. These should not be considered everyday clothing. They are for wearing when you go to the gym, or to yoga, or to a Nia, Pilates, or Zumba class.

Of course, when living with chronic illness, we want to be comfortable, but not at the expense of looking good. If nothing in your closet fits or is comfortable, and you've resorted to wearing pajamas or sportswear all day, every day, then it's time to do something about it. Most workout clothes aren't sexy unless you look like a model.

> " *There are 3 billion women who don't look like supermodels and only 8 who do."*
> - Anita Roddick, *The Body Shop*

What you wear has an impact on your self-esteem. Every time I walked past a mirror and saw myself—my face pale, unwashed hair, stretched-out yoga pants, and an old tee under a hoodie—I felt worse. Looking back, I now realize what I was looking at was a mixture of despair and self-pity. I couldn't deal with looking this way, so I'd walk away from the mirror and crawl back into bed.

Of course I wanted to do something about it, but didn't know where to begin, and didn't have the energy anyway. I was aware I was feeling a bit depressed, and when I mentioned it, one doctor offered me an anti-depressant. I said I'd think about it and let him know.

I felt that wasn't the right thing for me to do, but I wasn't sure if I could do anything else. I thought I would just have to feel, and look, like this until someone figured out how to fix me.

A FRESH START

There may not be much else you can do about the way you feel right this moment, but trust me - a shower, clean jeans or a nice pair of leggings and a soft shirt, some moisturizer on your face, and running a comb through your freshly-washed hair will make you feel better. Even if you have to sit on the floor in the shower, just get in there.

I don't know what spark finally made me crawl out of bed and decide to clean myself up, but I chose to look at it as a spiritual cleansing, too. It made me feel more capable, more alive.

Approach bathing as a ritual to wash off the day and to give yourself a fresh start. If you'd rather have a soak in the tub, do it. Many meds cause our skin to dry out, so stay hydrated inside and out with lots of water, and all-over moisturizer.

Afterward, if you need to, you can go lie down again, but try resting on the sofa. Give yourself a change of scenery. Take a nap if you need. Read a book - something on the best-seller list. Watch inspirational videos, or listen to motivational speakers. Avoid reality TV, and seek out things to lift your spirit, which will raise your vibration, and I promise you'll feel better.

KEEPING IT SIMPLE

Now that you've showered, let's find a few things to wear that afford you some color. When we are sick, we can lose our rosy glow. My complexion had a grayish-yellow tone to it because I became anemic. Not very pretty.

To counter those tones, I looked through my closet for shirts and tops in red and coral, blue and purple to brighten me up. I had them, but had forsaken them in favor of my favorite color - black. There'd be time for black later. Right now, I needed color! (Ignore your clothes in yellow, lime, gray, and pale pastel colors when you're sick. You need a big pop of color to look better and to raise your vibration.)

At some point I would have to go back to work, and as I lay there on the couch, I pondered what I would do about my clothes then. Some things to consider:

- ♥ What do you feel most comfortable in? (No, workout clothes don't count)
- ♥ Is there a dress code in your work environment?
- ♥ What would you love to wear if you were to change your style now?
- ♥ Do some of your clothes fit this ideal?

Look for a few outfits you enjoy wearing because they are comfortable and you know they look good on you. (For now, you only want what looks good and is comfortable) Do you need a couple things to pull everything together? A pair or two of black leggings? A longer-length sweater, or crisp tunic-length shirt, or floaty tops to wear over leggings? How about some sexy flats, or low chunky heels?

My goal was to simplify things, but I wanted to do it without getting so basic that there wasn't anything sexy about my clothes. I took pieces I loved, but which needed some work, and put them in a stack to take to a tailor. For instance - pants that were too long since I wasn't going to be wearing them with heels anymore. A beautiful shirt that needed darts to fit a little bit closer.

I liked a lot of my clothes, but I didn't have the energy to put together "outfits" any more, and the idea of suits tired me out just thinking about them. Some of my clothes were too fitted, and that felt exhausting. Others had buttons I couldn't button right now with my hands stiff and swollen.

I pictured myself wearing simple fitted maxi-dresses, wrap-dresses, and figure-flattering sheaths. Breezy skirts, and tops with great necklines, comfortable and stylish sandals and flats. Simple styles that can be easily dressed up or down, with jewelry, jackets, belts, and shoes.

And, of course, my jeans. Jeans are my uniform, always have been, so why fight it? They're what I'm most comfortable in, they fit me well, and they can be worn as both casual and dressy with the right shoes or boots, and top.

What are a couple of things you know you look and feel great in? Slowly put together more of those and eliminate all of the other things you just don't wear for one reason or another. Would more color be a good idea? Do you know your best colors? Ask your hair-stylist if you're not sure. In my experience, almost every woman looks great in jewel tones. Yellow is the only challenging one. Cool oranges and corals look great, too. Could a slightly sexier neckline be flattering?

What is your best feature? Play it up. Make your clothes work for you.

IN THE CLOSET

Marie Kondo's clothing clean-up is for when you're feeling better and ready to tackle a big, albeit fun, project. It will help get your wardrobe in alignment with how you intend to live your life from now on. Remember: Keeping it simple and sexy is the new black.

I spent a lot of time each morning standing and staring blankly at everything hanging in my closet, and finding nothing to wear. My tolerance for being uncomfortable had diminished greatly, so not much was appealing to me. I'd often look at my clothes and wonder what made me buy them.

When I finally tackled my closet to do a full "tidying," I found some clothes I loved, and lots of clothes I hadn't been ready to give away when we moved. This time, they went in my donation pile. I let them go knowing what clothes were left would fit, would look good, and would make me feel good about myself. And knowing I'd probably have fun doing a little bit of shopping.

I donated lots of shoes on my last closet clean-out, but kept a few pair that were so beautiful that I couldn't bear to give them up, even though I never wear them. I realize that's silly, so they went in my give-away pile this time.

Can you still comfortably wear all of your shoes? If not, give the ones that are in great shape to friends, or donate them. This is particularly important where high-heels are concerned. Achy joints and sky-high heels aren't a great combo, and not advisable for everyday wear because of what they do to our pelvis, knees, and spine, and the balls of our feet.

Here's a great rule for a pair of shoes: if you can't stride in them, give them up. There's nothing sexy about a woman hobbling along in a pair of too-high-for-her heels. Buy a lower, and just-as-stylish, pair. What you lose in the height will be made up for in your radiance.

I do have one caveat though: we should all have one amazing pair of heels, even if we can do nothing more than stagger from the closet to the bed. They can be great for our spirit!

An idea I recently saw suggested women have 9 pair of shoes. The example was: 3 pair of flats, 3 pair of heels of various heights, and three pair of boots. Athletic shoes would be included in flats, and in each group you would have a pair of casual, classic and dressy. I think 3 Casual + 3 Classic + 3 Dressy is a great idea for a place to start, and could be applied to our whole wardrobe.

With my closet done and my clothes in order, the last thing I did was address my dresser. I really think it's what I should have done first. Our bras, panties, and shape-wear are the foundation of all of our clothes. And, dare I say, our mental health? Bad bras can make great tops look bad. And think about this; if your panties don't fit well, or your undies are ugly, how sexy do you feel?

Get rid of granny-panties and old-lady functional bras. Buy a good nude bra (not white) that matches your skin-tone and a black one. These are your basics. Then throw in a sexy push-up in a pretty color, and perhaps a printed, silky, see-through. Done.

I found my lingerie drawer to be the most fun. I got rid of everything I didn't love and threw it all right into the trash bag. No regrets. Seven new pair of panties coming right up! They're so easy to order online. Bras are different; they need to be tried on for a perfect fit, so they were added to my shopping list. Everything is neat and visible now.

SOMETHING TO CONSIDER

If you haven't heard about "capsule wardrobes," it's an idea that gets floated out again every few years in fashion. The easy definition is that a capsule wardrobe is a minimal amount of clothing, say 20-30 pieces that mix-and-match and become a sort of uniform. Some women won't like the idea, wanting much more variety. But I like the idea as a place to start, especially when we aren't feeling well.

The appeal for me is not having to think about what to wear. Imagine: everything goes with everything else. It would save lots of energy, which is especially valuable when you don't have much, and leave it for other things that matter more. I've been looking at capsule wardrobes a lot on Pinterest lately.

Having only what you love in your closet, and having it all be comfortable, work together and flatter you, sounds like Heaven. Another perk is that less clothes equals less laundry, which equals more energy. Which adds up to feeling sexier.

THE TAKE-AWAY

Once you've cleaned out your closet and dresser, you have choices about what to do with those things. You can simply drop them at Goodwill or Salvation Army, of course. Or you can take them to a consignment shop that donates profits to a cause, or you can find a charity/thrift shop that helps women re-entering the workplace. You can take them to your church or donate them to recovery groups. You can deliver them to a haven for women who've had to flee their homes with only the clothes on their backs.

I never looked at it this way before, but cleaning and folding them is a way of expressing gratitude that these donated clothes have served you and will now serve someone new. Also, as you place the ones you are throwing out in a trash bag, thank them for keeping you clothed all of this time. Both are a lovely way to maintain that attitude of gratitude.

KISS AND MAKE-UP

"Nope, this won't do," is what I said to myself most mornings as I stood looking in the mirror. In an effort to get some color back into my face I used under-eye cover cream, foundation and powdered blush, and topping it all off with a mineral powder.

It both felt and looked like a mask. And after all the effort I put into my hair, it was hanging limply before I'd even left the bathroom. It was clear I needed a new way to look good without using every bit of energy on my changing hair and paler complexion.

I didn't have the option of going to work without being pulled together - not when it's my job to make others look and feel great. And if I didn't look great, I certainly couldn't go in looking as bad as I felt. I thought about the conversation I would have with a client sitting in my chair facing this same challenge:

- ♥ Right now we need to make over your hair and make-up. Then see what happens later.
- ♥ How much energy do you have to achieve a new look daily?
- ♥ How open are you to great new ideas?
- ♥ Then I'd offer solutions that I felt would best help her achieve her goals.

Now, I asked that of myself. When I got right down to it, my goal was to look better than I felt, and to be able to accomplish it easily. I don't think that's asking too much. (Although on some days it almost is.) Those are the days I am grateful I took stock of the situation, made the necessary changes, and created a simple beauty routine for myself.

> " *Be as simple as you can be; you will be astonished to see how uncomplicated and happy your life can become.*"
>
> - Paramahansa Yogananda

CROWNING GLORY

First things first - I started with my hair. I'd never had to spend much time on my hair because it was beautiful curls. Now it has become thinner, fragile, and less curly because of the medicines. I feel best, sexiest, and can easily manage my hair when it's cut quite short. I went through a variety of shorter cuts and finally settled on an individualized pixie cut, adding a rich, red color.

You too must find a cut that is easy and flattering with very little work. A cut that works with your hair's density and texture, as well as with your bone-structure. An unwashed ponytail is not a solution. Neither are inch-long roots. Talk with your stylist about a lower-maintenance cut and color routine until you are feeling better. You will be surprised at all of the options they can offer!

Changing my color to a red worked beautifully with my paler complexion. If you color your hair at home, ask a friend if the color is still flattering. I will say, a little golden tone or warmth (red) can perk us up when we feel ill and washed out. They are also more youthful.

Also make a commitment to do your touch-up regularly, and do it properly by only touching-up the new growth. Put your hair on your calendar and keep your appointment. Commit to yourself because "roots" aren't sexy.

LET'S FACE IT

Our skin often becomes dehydrated when we are not well. Depending on our illness, we can become pale. I was pale, and it wasn't a pretty pale, either. I looked more vampire-victim than creamy vixen. To add insult to injury, not only was I dealing with illness and medicines, but my age had affected my skin, too. I needed an expert opinion, so I took my concerns to a longtime friend who is a sought-after makeup artist. Best. Advice. Ever.

♥ She told me not to try and compensate for my pallor with an opaque foundation. She recommended using a tinted moisturizer or BB cream. If I really needed a foundation, use something very sheer and lightweight. (Note: Always be sure there is an SPF 15-30.)

♥ Next, she suggested I change to a cream blush since powder blushes show every wrinkle. A warm pink is a good color for most everyone. I chose one just for its name, Orgasm, and love it. The blush and its matching lipstick always bring a smile to my face when I get ready!

♥ Last, she suggested finishing with a sheer mineral powder in the palest pink to give me a bit of tint and sparkle. It's her signature touch on her special occasion make-up, making brides look soft and radiant.

Now my morning makeup routine is as easy as one-two-three:

1. I apply BB cream (summer) or sheer foundation (winter) with a damp makeup sponge.
2. I add a dab of cream blush at the apples of my cheeks, which I gently blend down toward my ears with my fingers.
3. I brush on my soft mineral powder and my skin looks great in under five minutes!

THE EYES HAVE IT

I always fill in my brows since they too have become thinner. I always told my clients to do this too, because eyes without eyebrows are like a beautiful painting without a frame. If you aren't sure how to do your brows or what to use, ask at any make-up counter. They will gladly show you how, and find the perfect-for-you product, making it easy to apply and stay put. Good products will last a year or two.

I complimented a woman on her brows once, and she told me she had been frustrated because she couldn't make her brows identical. When she mentioned this to her make-up artist, he told her, "Honey, your brows are sisters, but they're NOT identical twins!" Symmetry only exists where Botox has gone before.

If you are lucky enough to have full eyebrows, but shaping them is a challenge and you always end up looking more Vulcan than Vogue, have the esthetician at your salon do your brows. Turn yourself over to her skilled hands, and then keep your hands off. One of my sisters (not mentioning names here) used to work on her brows until there was nothing left but a little bitty comma. Don't be like her.

I don't have the energy to deal with mascara that runs, so I always use black waterproof mascara. Doing my brows and adding mascara takes minutes at most. I can take another few minutes and apply a couple of quick sweeps of eye shadow.

I keep my palette natural looking, and use pigment-packed colors that compliment my eye color - not my clothes. And last, I add eyeliner. Bobbi Brown said, "The best thing a woman can do is to learn to draw a thin black line of eyeliner on her top lid." It's elegant, makes eyes look more open, and lashes look thicker. (Trust me: Never line only the bottom lid, the visual weight of it pulls your whole face down.)

If I only did one thing to my face, I'd apply a tinted-sunscreen.
If I did two things, I'd add mascara.
Three things would be my tinted-sunscreen, lashes, and finish my brows.
One more? Lip tint with sunscreen.
If you have more energy, go have fun!

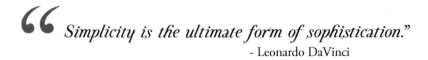 *Simplicity is the ultimate form of sophistication."*
- Leonardo DaVinci

SIMPLIFY, SIMPLIFY, SIMPLIFY

When I was recovering from my first flare-up, I couldn't hold a pencil, a pen, or a make-up brush. When I felt better, I looked for makeup brushes with larger handles that would be helpful for women with arthritis or other joint issues, and found beautiful bamboo brush sets with thicker handles. Size does matter; don't let anyone tell you otherwise!

To streamline my daily routine, I discarded all of the extraneous hair care, skin care, and makeup products and samples that cluttered my makeup bag and cabinet. What's the point of a 32-color eye shadow palette when I only use four of the colors consistently? Yes, it was pretty, and I had paid for it, but it was useless. As were all of the foundations, blushes, and bronzers that no longer worked with my skin tone, and all of the mousses, gels, and hairspray I hoped would make my hair behave again.

I let it all go.

My shower stall got a makeover, too. Commercial bar soaps dried out my skin unless they were creamy, but then they left a film on both my skin and my shower. The shower became slippery when wet, and chalky looking when dry, which meant more work to clean it. I don't need more work, and I bet you don't either. Now I use a natural, clear body-wash on my skin, or else I use a glycerin soap (which can't sit in water - it melts).

Unfortunately, some of my perfumes no longer smelled nice on me. Have you noticed that, too? Since I never wore them anymore, I gave them away, leaving myself with two perfumes that smell great and make me feel pampered.

THE TAKE-AWAY

Keeping it simple and sexy has paid off. I have less clutter in my bathroom and it's easy to keep clean and organized. An antique silver tray, a previously unused heirloom, now holds cottonballs and Q-tips in glass jars next to my perfumes.

My makeup fits in one cosmetics bag, my hair care fits in a plastic box, and first-aid products are in another under the sink. Not rummaging around makes my morning routine quick and easy, saving much-needed energy. Which has the added benefit of making me feel better, which makes me look better.

KISS mission accomplished!

GET SOME SLEEP

If I had to be one of the seven dwarfs, I'd most like to be Happy. More often than not, I'm either Grumpy or Sleepy. What I know about getting a good night's sleep could fit on the back of a cocktail napkin. No, make that a business card. I've had trouble sleeping ever since I developed the first illness in 1998.

It's not like I'm "scrub the bathroom tile with a toothbrush" wide-awake. I just can't get to sleep. And I don't understand why when I feel so flipping tired, I can't just lie down, close my eyes, and wake up tomorrow.

Now I understand why my infant son would fuss and cry when he was over-tired. I'd pat his back, rock his crib, play music for him, and if all of that failed to soothe, I'd pick him up and pace the floors with him. The family dog, Samantha, pacing with me the whole time.

As I walked in circles, I wondered why he didn't just fall sleep. I wonder that same thing now, lying in bed watching the ceiling fan spinning, and listening to cars going somewhere at 3:00 a.m. Where are they going at this hour? Why aren't they in bed? Why am I still awake?

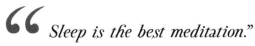
Sleep is the best meditation."
- Dalai Lama

Since our bodies repair and rebuild themselves while we sleep, getting enough sleep is vital. What's enough sleep, you ask? Anywhere from seven to nine hours, depending on your body's own needs.

How much sleep do you usually get?

Getting as little as one extra hour of sleep a night can be beneficial to your health, mood, weight, and even your sex life.

Let's start with that reason for getting enough sleep: increased libido. Upwards of one-quarter of the population says their sex lives suffer because they're just too tired.

Sound familiar? Our levels of both estrogen and testosterone are lower when we are sleep deprived. So, a bit more sleep will have you feeling a bit sexier, and that's a good thing.

Studies also found that too little sleep is linked to serious health problems, such as increased risk for certain cancers and faster tumor growth, heart disease and heart attacks, diabetes, and obesity. People who sleep less than seven hours a night were almost 3X more likely to catch a cold as people who sleep eight hours or more a night. We don't need an increased risk of catching every bug that comes around.

Another great reason to get enough sleep is that our metabolism works more efficiently when we get enough sleep. When we are always tired, our metabolism slows down in an effort to preserve energy.

Also, when we're tired, we're more likely to skip our exercise class, or to skip preparing a healthy meal for ourselves. Without enough sleep, leptin levels drop, and leptin, another hormone, plays a key role in making us feel full. Feeling exhausted can make junk food seem more acceptable, and then hitting the couch is an easier option than hitting the gym.

If you are one of the women living with chronic pain, getting enough sleep may actually make you hurt less and reduce your need for pain medication. Recent studies linked less sleep to a lower pain threshold.

Ironically, pain often makes it harder to get the sleep you need. Be sure you're doing everything you can to address your pain: exercise, yoga, meditation, massage, hot bath, relaxation CDs, and if necessary, pain relievers with a sleep aid.

> **"** *On days when I'm tired, everything seems to be too much to deal with. When I'm well-rested, I can tackle just about anything."*
> — Donna O'Klock

You'll be in a better mood when you get enough sleep. It won't guarantee a Little Miss Sunshine disposition all of the time, but I'm sure you've realized that when you feel exhausted, you're also more likely to be a little bitchy or short-tempered. In "doctor speak," that lack of sleep affects our emotional regulation.

Not getting enough sleep also affects how we think by impairing comprehension, affecting our ability to pay attention, and having an impact on our decision-making abilities. It can also make us accident-prone - we are more likely to trip, or cut ourselves while cooking, and it can also result in distracted driving.

Some days I have more trouble with my memory, and I attributed it to my age or the meds, but sleep loss can also lead to forgetfulness. During sleep our brains process and consolidate memories from the day. By not getting enough sleep, there's a chance those memories might not get stored correctly - or get lost.

> **"** *Let her sleep for when she wakes, she will move mountains."*
> — Unknown

If you also have trouble getting a great night's sleep, here are a few things to do:

♥ WHEN you go to sleep is as important as how much sleep you get. Aim for 7 to 9 hours a night. Studies show you'll feel more rested if you sleep from 10 p.m. until 6:00 a.m. rather than getting eight hours from midnight to 8:00 a.m.

♥ Set a schedule and stick to it. If you know you enjoy reading for 30 minutes, factor that in, and go to bed earlier. Aim for LIGHTS OUT at the same time each night to reinforce your body's wake-sleep cycle.

♥ Removing makeup, applying moisturizer, brushing and flossing, dental guards, nighttime meds, even taking a warm shower, all ease our transition from busyness to restfulness. Build this into your nighttime SCHEDULE so you can have the lights out on time.

♥ Turn off the TV and ELECTRONICS a little earlier. Growing evidence has come to light that electronic devices interfere with our sleep. I've been listening to classical music as a way to wind down before bed. I've also gone back to reading paper books at night.

♥ It seemed that the moment I'd lie down, everything I couldn't remember until JUST THIS MINUTE popped into my head. I've found that sitting down and JOURNALING before bed is also a good way of emptying my head. My monkey-mind feels acknowledged, and leaves me alone to sleep.

♥ Food and Beverage Department: don't go to bed hungry, but don't go to bed on a full stomach, either. Pay attention to how much CAFFEINE you have in the late afternoon. And although ALCOHOL may make you feel sleepy initially, it will interrupt your sleep later in the night, so enjoy responsibly.

♥ Using a diffuser in your bedroom is also a delicious way to relax. Use natural ESSENTIAL OILS. Lavender oil is always what comes to my mind first, but chamomile, sandalwood, neroli, and ylang-ylang are also calming oils. Find one that is sensual and pleasing. And if you share a bedroom, one that pleases your partner, too.

" *There is a time for many words, and there is also a time for sleep.*"

- Homer

SECTION 2

THE BENEFITS OF JOURNALING

There are many reasons to keep a journal.

It's useful to keep track of what's going on with new meds, or when trying things out, such as dietary changes. I've seen patterns unfold over time by looking back in my journals. It helps me remember things I want to discuss with my doctors, or a question that popped into my mind in the middle of the night, if I have written them down in the journal.

Sometimes my daily journaling is nothing more than a bitch session, where I let it all hang out; I've written about job issues, co-workers, clients. I've bitched about family stuff, money stuff, the insurance company, test results, and relationship issues.

A journal is a good place to put my fears to get them outside of myself, rather than have them roiling inside of me. It can be a way of taking out the trash, and if you want to, you can rip out that page and burn it, let it go. Gone, girl. If you looked at my journal, you'd see the ragged edges where many pages were torn out to be burned.

Our fears are reasonable and worth exploring, there's nothing sexy about denial, and it's better to get it all out than hold any of it in. Sometimes, when venting on the page, I suddenly see the error in my logic. I see where I was flat wrong and need to change the way I'm looking at something. I love it when I'm able to get some perspective, and gain a little altitude on my attitude. Or when I find the right words to say to someone. Or find the courage to say the words I've been feeling.

I have been journaling for more than 24 years - I began in earnest when I bought

Julia Cameron's life-changing book, *The Artist's Way*, and started using her tool, Morning Pages: writing three pages, longhand, every morning for 12 weeks. Great stuff has come out of those pages.

I've always known journaling was good not only for my head, my attitude, and my creativity, but also for my health. I could make myself feel better by sitting down and writing. Didn't matter what it was, just that I sat down and wrote for a while.

Now professionals acknowledge these ideas, with increasing evidence to support the idea that journaling has a positive impact on physical well-being. James Pennebaker, a UT Austin psychologist and researcher, asserts that regular journaling strengthens immune cells, called T-lymphocytes. He believes "writing about stressful events helps you come to terms with them, thus reducing their impact on your physical health."

Yet another great reason to go buy yourself a beautiful journal and start writing.

HOW TO JOURNAL

Journaling is simply writing down your thoughts and feelings. Doing it regularly helps you establish a commitment to yourself. I've done it for so long that I find that I automatically relax when I sit to journal. It's beneficial if you are feeling anxious, stressed or depressed, since it can help you gain some clarity or perspective about why you are feeling that way.

I learned to trust myself more by making the commitment to journal. Keeping promises to ourselves is especially important when we are chronically ill. Why? Because it's important to know that no matter what, you are there for yourself. You will do what's best for you. That you are on your side. You'd be surprised how many women don't have this faith in themselves. It's important to our well-being.

TOOLS

You don't need a luxury notebook - unless you want one, or it would make journaling feel more special as you establish your routine.

I have written on hundreds of Office Depot legal pads, (I'm partial to their purple paper) and in composition notebooks, great because I'm a lefty and there are no rings or spirals in my way. I've written in hand-made journals, leather-bound journals, and even, when desperate, awkwardly scrawled in spiral-bound school notebooks from Target.

You don't need a fancy pen, but I've had a few of them through the years. You just want ink that doesn't smear. Or you can use a pencil, which I like because I can erase when I make a mistake. They also don't fade like ink does over time. According to the National Archives, "graphite pencil is a very stable material that does not fade in light and doesn't bleed in water." I don't really care about my journals surviving forever, every few years I throw them out anyway.

Whichever tool you choose needs to fit your hand comfortably. There is a connection between the act of writing and the fact that it stimulates the RAS - Reticular Activating System - in our brain, giving importance to what we are focusing on in that moment. Handwriting also prevents us from being distracted, which keeps us sharper all the way around.

Journaling is simple: sit down, pen in hand, paper in front of you, and start.

Try writing in short, focused bursts - say 20 minutes at a time. Give yourself a prompt if you need one:

- ♥   I can't think of a thing to say -
- ♥   I feel terrible today because -
- ♥   I feel great today because -
- ♥   I am so scared that -
- ♥   Every time I eat this -
- ♥   I'm so pleased that -
- ♥   What if? -
- ♥   I feel unlovable because -
- ♥   I feel so loved because -
- ♥   I hope that -

& Sexy

- ♥ It would be great if -
- ♥ I have this interesting idea -
- ♥ Good news! -
- ♥ I am grateful that -
- ♥ I am so excited -
- ♥ I realized that -

Nobody says you have to journal at home; take yourself to a nearby coffeehouse, bakery, library, bookstore, or park and just revel in having some time alone to think, dream, and write. You don't need to do it alone, either. Meet a friend who is also journaling and work together. Set a timer for your writing and afterward you can catch up and share.

What sexier way to find out what is inside of you, to organize your thoughts, or to observe your progress, than by taking some uninterrupted quiet time each day and writing in your journal?

AH, INERTIA

In any situation, the best thing you can do is the right thing; the next best thing you can do is the wrong thing; the worst thing you can do is nothing."

- Theodore Roosevelt

I was thinking about inertia the other day when I was having trouble motivating myself to get up, put on my Adidas, and go outside and pretend to be an athlete. I was trying to convince myself to go for a walk, and I hate to admit it, but I never did go for that walk.

And here I am again today, feeling overwhelmingly tired. I assume you know what I mean when I say that I feel like I've run out of juice. Or as if my batteries have completely run down. Or I feel unplugged. The worst thing for me to do is to keep avoiding that walk. But I've lost my superpowers, and Inertia has become my nemesis.

I have a cartoon pinned above my desk: a girl sitting on her bed in her gym clothes, the caption reads, "Damn, I didn't make it to the gym today. That makes five years

& Sexy

in a row!" The first time I saw it, I laughed until tears streamed down my face.

This is from my 24-year-old *American Heritage Dictionary*, on Inertia:

1. A tendency to do nothing or to remain unchanged.
2. A property of matter by which it continues in its existing state of rest.
3. Indisposition to motion, exertion, or change.

I love the last definition, because I have felt completely indisposed to moving or exerting myself in any way, and I didn't see it changing anytime in the near future. You probably remember this from high school - in its simplest form the principle of inertia states that, "A body in motion tends to stay in motion, and a body at rest tends to stay at rest." There have been so many times I have thought, "If only there were a battery-charger I could plug into and feel energized, full of vitality!"

Well, there's good news and there's bad news. The good news: there is! The bad news: it's called exercise.

Not what you wanted to hear, I know.

Since becoming ill, I've realized exercise is one of the most important things we can all do to build, or rebuild, a joyful, healthy, and sexy life! Physical movement gets everything else moving, too. Our spirits lift when we overcome our inertia. Our color improves as we get our circulation going. Getting moving makes us feel better about things and better about ourselves.

My self-esteem rises because not only did I intend to do something, I did it. Movement creates momentum, and momentum is exactly what we need.

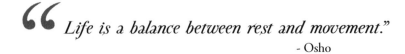

> **"** *Life is a balance between rest and movement."*
> - Osho

Sometimes we haven't moved meaningfully in so long that we can't imagine what our first step should be. We have been a body at rest (okay, I'm talking about myself here) and it would be so much easier to continue doing nothing than to exert ourselves.

With all of these thoughts in mind, I called my dearest friend, Holly Curtis-Nastasi, M.Ed. and Black Belt Nia Educator, to ask for her advice on how to get going again once we've found ourselves at a standstill.

I met Holly 24 years ago in a personal-growth seminar led by Robert Kiyosaki, co-author of *Rich Dad, Poor Dad*. Holly was an aerobics instructor, and a runner, back then. She was also the only woman I'd ever met who could do a one-armed push-up. We became friends, and started running together. She taught classes for many years, and like other aerobics teachers, complained of the pains and aches that came along with high-impact exercise.

At an industry convention, she discovered a new aerobic movement technique, met the creators, and fell in love with them, their ideas, and their classes. Not long after, she went to Portland for training, and when she returned she stopped teaching impact aerobics, quit running, and switched to exclusively teaching the Nia Technique. I became her first student (a very willing guinea pig) as she learned to teach the grounded movements and dynamic ease that Nia offered.

Fast forward to present day: Holly is STILL teaching her own Nia classes and traveling to teach the teachers, and she is a highly anticipated guest-teacher everywhere she visits. She loves sharing the joy that movement can bring every body.

I rely on her expertise and often call her for inspiration and motivation. Movement is as important to our overall health as breathing - we are designed to move in order to keep our body functioning properly. And movement becomes especially important when we live with chronic illness and we always feel tired, because it will make us feel less tired.

A journey of a thousand miles begins with a single step."

- Lao Tzu

After months and months, I finally called and asked Holly if she had any suggestions to make it easier to get up off the couch and get started moving again. What would be the best thing for me, or anyone in this situation, to do? What would be a great first step? Here is what Holly had to say:

Q - How do we even begin to move when we feel this exhausted?

A - You know what I'd suggest, first thing? Get down on the floor and roll around, wallow in the sensation. See what happens and how you feel when you get back up. That's what Nia is all about, reveling in the sensations in the body.

Q - When you are chronically tired, why should you consider exercising?

A - To offer yourself relief from achiness. And to find out what would make you feel better.

Q – But how do I overcome this inertia?

A – Just "kick-start" it. Make yourself do something. Put some music on and dance in your kitchen. Go for a walk. Attend a class. Think of movement as something that you're going to get a reward from RIGHT NOW - not as some big future goal that's out there.

Q - But won't exercise make me feel more tired?

A - Experiment. See how a little exercise makes you feel. Do this and see how you feel. Do you feel just a little bit better? Now do that, and see how you feel. Did that make you feel a little bit better? When you experiment like this, remind yourself, I'm going to do this because I will feel better right now. Don't push yourself, just ease into it.

Q – What else can you add for us about overcoming inertia?

A - Just like a car, the hardest part is getting it moving again once it's stopped. It takes more gas to get it going again than it takes to keep it going.
And just like that car, once you're in motion, you will pick up energy. Remember, every day isn't going to be exactly like the next one, or like the last. Enjoy what's there for you each day. Stay present. Stay in the now.

It seems like a stretch to think about enjoying movement when you feel like this, right? But to enjoy what's there for you, start by doing something easy to accomplish. Afterward, check in with yourself and see how it made you feel. Tell yourself something positive about what you just did.

It can be even be this simple: if you've been on the couch all day, get up and make a cup of tea, grab a piece of fruit, put it all on a tray and carry it outside to enjoy. If you can't do that, find a nice place to sit and enjoy your treat. You've gone from a prone position, to moving around your kitchen, and now you are sitting (outside in the fresh air) with a treat. Find pleasure in this moment, and remind yourself how good it is to be able to do this for yourself.

This could be your starting point – it could lead to getting up and putting on your sneakers and taking a short stroll down the street tomorrow. Be careful, you might find yourself saying "Hello" to a neighbor, petting someone's cat, talking to a dog through a fence, and stopping to smell the flowers along the way.

HOMO ERECTUS

When we keep focusing all of our attention inward on how bad we feel, we will keep feeling bad. We contract energetically. But when we get up and focus our attention outward, we allow our reality to expand. We notice the world is still there, still beautiful, and still waiting for us to participate.

Here are some more ways to get moving that will remind you how good movement actually feels:

- ♥ Follow Holly's suggestion - lie down on the floor and move around a bit. Roll. Stretch. Contract. Gently pull your knees to your chest. Follow what you are inspired to do.

- ♥ Put some music on and let it encourage you to wiggle, sway, cha-cha, or dance freely.

- ♥ I love my exercise ball. I can bounce on it. I can also stretch by draping over it, and it's comfortable for sitting for long periods of time.

♥ Put on flip-flops and go for a little "mosey." Set a casual goal, just to the end of the block and back.

♥ Put on your sneakers and head out the door for a stroll. Take some music. Take a friend. Take the dog. Take the kids. Make it a parade!

♥ Buy yourself a yoga CD and mat. Start easy, then when you have more energy and more confidence, you can go to a class.

♥ Get a Hula Hoop. You're smiling, aren't you? If you have kids, borrow theirs, if not, buy one in your favorite color. Hooping breaks the monotony of walking or biking, and can improve core strength and spinal mobility. They burn calories while improving balance and coordination. Best of all, they're fun!

♥ Take a Nia class. Nia is perfect for every body at every movement level. The music is always great, and the teachers always delightful, no matter where in the country I take a class.

♥ Take a bicycle ride. Feel the freedom of moving forward, wind in your face.

♥ If you have one available, walk on a treadmill, or ride a stationary bike. Start slow, add great music.

♥ Get in a pool. The buoyancy is wonderful for aching joints. If you're up for swimming laps, do it. Swimming is the best form of non-impact exercise.

♥ Rowing. Kayaking. Stand-up Paddle-boards. You can now find classes pretty much everywhere there's water.

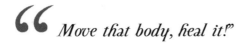 *Move that body, heal it!"*

-Professor Trance

Here's my last thought on movement and dealing with feeling tired - it's so easy to keep telling ourselves that we are on the couch all day because we are tired. But it's closer to the truth to say we are tired because we have been on the couch all day.

Overcoming inertia is yet another example of "fake it till you make it." You have to suit-up and show up, go and do things as if you have the energy, and know eventually you will have more energy.

Ease Through Exercise

There are so many ways to move and to get exercise that are beneficial to both our bodies and our minds. We talked about easy ways to get going in the chapter on INERTIA. But, the very first step starts in your head, by making up your mind that exercise is something you will make time for because it will make you feel better.

And because if you don't take care of yourself… you can't take care of anyone else.

As we get moving, we will gain strength and confidence, and eventually mastery. We can also enjoy the process every step of the way. It's important to choose the right type of exercise for where you are right now, not where you wish you were. When you can barely climb a flight of stairs, wanting to party to Pitbull at a Zumba class isn't going to be the right fit.

You may want to take a gentle yoga class, or start by taking an easy walk every day, adding a bit more time and distance as the days go by. This will get you moving, give you energy, and get you back out in the world. Let it be easy and pleasurable.

Most of the complaints people attribute to either getting older, or to their illnesses, are really just an effect of their sedentary lifestyle.

When I got sick and tired of feeling sick and tired and ready to get moving again, I began going for short walks. I used to call it "taking a mosey," and to be sure I didn't push myself, I moseyed in my flip-flops.

I also began using a gentle yoga video at home. When I could do the whole class easily, I began attending yoga classes at a nearby studio. It felt wonderful to be out among people again. Eventually I built up to walking for 45 minutes a couple of times a week and taking yoga flow classes. It didn't happen overnight, but it did happen.

> " *Lack of activity destroys the good condition of every human being, while movement and methodical physical exercise save it and preserve it.*"
>
> - Plato

Do you spend your time at a desk all week, then come home exhausted? Then try a gentle yoga class, a yoga-nidra class, or one marked as suitable for beginners. The gentle movements will help you to stretch-out your body, and calm your mind.

Is your back your weak spot, literally? Joints ache? Try swimming at a neighborhood pool or your local Y. The buoyancy of water is good for your body and joints, countering gravity's pull. We began our lives in warm water, and there's a lot to be said for its ability to soothe and nurture us.

If you have the energy, Pilates is a wonderful way to strengthen our core muscles, taking us from hunched and exhausted to erect, strong, and comfortable. Look for beginner's classes on their machines with a personal instructor, and mat classes both privately and in a group.

Like the idea of lifting weights? I do, too. Load-bearing exercise is good for building strong muscles and maintaining strong bones. This is one exercise that pays high dividends right now, and later in life for women. Now, I feel good about wearing sleeveless dresses since my arms are toned. And feeling strong translates into how capable I feel dealing with illness, and with life in general. Later on: weightlifting will keep my bones strong and help me avoid fractures.

Work up to aerobic classes after being ill for any length of time. What fun is a class when you can't breathe, or feel weak in the knees or dizzy? One of the best things about Nia classes is that they are for everybody at any level. You will see people moving slowly and gently, while others are working hard. It's all good!

Whatever you choose, start slowly, stay open-minded, enjoy being a beginner. Choose any type of aerobic activity that feels like fun and lifts your spirits.

> " *To keep the body in good health is a duty - otherwise we shall not be able to keep our mind strong and clear."*
>
> - Buddha

When I began lifting weights, I treated it as only a means to an end. I wasn't going to enjoy it until I had the results I wanted: six-pack abs, a tight butt, and definition in my arms and legs.

Soon I was thinking about quitting because I wasn't having any fun. One morning I realized I wasn't letting it be fun. I needed to find a way to enjoy myself in order to stay with it long enough to get hooked. I learned to enjoy the process, and to find pleasure and sensuality in the movement.

I also made a couple of great playlists on my iPod, to reinforce that idea, and from that point forward, I listened to music as I warmed up on the treadmill, and then moved over to lift weights. I started with baby steps and was amazed that over the course of just a month, I could lift twice as much as when I began. One more month and my arms already looked good. By removing my conditions, I had fun. Each time I went to the gym, I celebrated myself. It's important to acknowledge ourselves when we keep our commitments to fitness.

Here's the $50 Million Dollar Question that we must all ask: If I don't take care of my body now, what will my quality of life be like later?" To answer that question, all we need do is look around.

As Debbie Rosas, the creator of Nia says, "Through movement we find health." She should know. She's been living, and moving bodies, in meaningful ways for almost forty years.

Through movement we will be able to live our lives with more ease, grace, health, and confidence. Are you looking for a class yet?

YOGA BEGINS WITH A "WHY?"

If you already go to the gym, or walk or run regularly, you've probably created a routine that you enjoy. Why would you want to add yoga? If you're too tired, or if you have arthritis, a bad shoulder, bad knees, or a bad back, why would you want go to a yoga class? (Note - Please don't call your body parts "bad," it hurts their feelings.)

Why should anyone take a yoga class? What would it change? In one word — everything!

❝ *Yoga teaches us to cure what need not be endured and endure what cannot be cured."*

- B.K. Iyengar

I have always seen myself as more of a mover, dancer, gym-goer, but every time I take a yoga class, I've left feeling peaceful, relaxed, and pain-free. And each time I ask myself, "Why don't I do this more often?"

I promised myself when we moved I would do yoga at a studio nearby. After reviewing their class schedule, and description of each class, I chose a class. It had been a few years and now that I had a chronic illness, I could barely keep up. But

I didn't throw in the towel. I went back and tried a Yin Yoga class. With no idea what to expect, despite having read the description, I let go of any expectations and focused on the teacher's silky voice as she guided the class.

Breathe in, now breathe out. Find traction. Allow. Allow. Allow.

During one long pose lying on my back, my whole body was relaxed, except for my right shoulder, which was so tight that I kept wiggling. The teacher silently came over, placed a small sandbag on my shoulder and surprisingly, my shoulder let go. My whole body immediately relaxed and tears streamed down my face. I lay there with tears filling my ears, releasing all of the tension that had been building for who-knows-how-long?

At my third class, again Yin Yoga, the teacher spoke about the synovial joints in our bodies – found in the elbows, wrists, thumbs, shoulders, hips, knees, neck, and feet. The inner synovial membrane secretes lubricating, shock absorbing, and joint-nourishing synovial fluid. These joints receive nutrition from the surrounding blood supply in a process achieved best through exercise. And the long, slow poses of yoga are the perfect way to nurture these joints.

Nurturing our joints is beneficial, no matter our age, if we want to become, or stay, flexible. And if your chronic illness is one that affects your joints, this is of extra importance. You know the old saying, "If you don't use it, you lose it." This applies to our joints and our mobility, too. (Check with your doctor before trying a new exercise class.)

YOGA NIDRA

Yoga Nidra is something I'd only recently experienced, and now I do it at least three times a week. As my friend Gina Waterfield prepared to teach her first yoga nidra class, she invited me. "You've got to come try this, it will make you feel so good."

She wasn't kidding.

Yoga Nidra is called the yoga of aware sleep. For those of us who feel chronically exhausted, it's one of the deepest states of relaxation we can be in without being asleep, and it's a systematic way to address our body, mind, and subconscious-mind's needs. It decreased my stress and tension immediately, and I felt happy and rejuvenated later.

During our class, Gina encouraged us to get as comfortable as we could, as if we were building a nest. Then we covered up snugly. Speaking in soft tones, Gina guided us to bring awareness to different parts of our body. We worked our way systematically through our body and into a deep state of relaxation. Then she led us back to waking, and yoga nidra was brought to a close. Yoga Nidra is different than traditional yoga classes - it's a mini-retreat.

Now, when I haven't sleep well, I fit a 30-minute session (available online for free) into my afternoon. Doing so gives me a boost of energy in a healthy, refreshing way, instead of having a cup of coffee, which keeps my poor-sleep cycle going.

Yoga nidra feels like an act of deepest self-nurturing. Find a class so you can experience it at least once.

> ❝ *Yoga allows you to find an inner peace that is not ruffled and riled by the endless stresses and struggles of life.*❞
>
> - B.K. Iyengar

GREAT REASONS TO BEGIN DOING YOGA:

1. No matter which yoga class you decide to take, there are movements perfect for every level of student.

2. It's an ideal way to get in touch, and fall in love, with your body. I hear many women speak badly about their bodies, especially when they're ill. Support your body, and in return, it will support you with increased strength and flexibility.

3. Yoga will improve your posture. Our heads are as heavy as a bowling ball. When balanced over a nice, straight spine it takes less effort to support it and we stand taller. This helps us to look better than we often feel. If you sit at a desk all day, yoga will help you uncurl and breathe better, which aids in our circulation and stress management.

4. Yoga can improve sleep by easing the pain symptoms in those with arthritis, back pain, fibromyalgia, and other chronic conditions. Reduced pain increases our chances of a better night's sleep.

5. It helps with IBS and constipation. Yoga, like most types of exercise, can ease constipation through movement. My yoga teacher/massage therapist friend always called the twisting poses a "massage for your guts."

6. Yoga develops our physical and mental strength. The stretches and poses aid muscle development, increase core strength, help maintain our nervous system, improve our balance, and release tension in our limbs. The focused breathing can improve our lung capacity. Staying in the moment clears our mind, which decreases stress and improves our mental health.

7. And mental strength may be the best benefit of yoga. The same discipline that fuels a consistent yoga practice will help overcome inertia and change habits that no longer serve us, developing new habits that will.

When you look at all of yoga's benefits, you'll notice everything is connected, and this feeds the upward spiral of wellness. And that upward spiral will lift us back up to feeling sexy again!

Rubbed the Right Way

I could simply say, "Go for massages," but I want to show you all of the reasons behind what I've learned from direct experience. Massage has been a regular part of my life for more than 25 years. I used to have one monthly when I was a busy hairstylist; they were a necessity since I stood still, arms and shoulders raised all day. They helped my body stay strong and flexible, and my muscles stay relaxed. A massage was good for my circulation, my lymphatic system, and most especially, my spirit.

> **"** *Massage has had a positive effect on every medical condition we've looked at."*
>
> - Tiffany Field, Ph.D.

I am glad massage has become mainstream and is now recognized as a part of complementary and alternative medicine. Mayo Clinic studies have found it may be helpful for digestive disorders, myofascial pain syndrome, parasthesia and nerve pain, and TMJ pain. Massage can ease the distress caused by migraines. It's especially effective on lower back and neck and shoulder pain. A massage can help with the tenderness that results from fibromyalgia, and it can help to prevent PMS and reduce its symptoms, such as mood swings, cramps, and water retention.

I read an article from the NIH Center for Complementary and Alternative Medicine which said, "The benefits may last as long as a year after just a few treatments."

While they've not lasted that long for me, I usually feel better immediately, and that comfort usually lasts from one visit to the next. When I don't wait until I am in pain, I feel progressively better with each massage, and I feel better between each visit.

> " *Effective health care depends on self-care;*
> *this fact is currently heralded as if it were a*
> *discovery.*"
>
> – Ivan Illich

Studies show that massage reduces levels of the stress hormone cortisol, while boosting levels of serotonin and dopamine (our feel-good hormones). By doing this, massage slows our heart rate, reduces blood pressure, and blocks the nervous system's pain receptors. By increasing blood flow to muscles, it may even help them heal. Reduced levels of cortisol have been shown to give our immune system a boost, even in people with severely compromised immune systems.

As you saw in the chapter on Pleasure, doing things that feel good results in great benefits for both our body and our health.

It's also been observed that massage decreases activity in the right lobe of our brain, which is more active when we're sad, and increases functioning in the left lobe, which is activated when we're happy. Dr. Andrew Weil states, "Massage therapy has been shown to relieve depression, especially in people who have chronic fatigue syndrome."

Massage also increases delta waves - the brain waves associated with deep sleep, which is why it is so easy to fall asleep on the massage table. I usually fall asleep, only to wake in a puddle of drool. As often as it happens, you'd think I wouldn't be embarrassed any more, but I still am. My sweet massage therapist always laughs, saying, "Most of my clients fall asleep, and they all drool."

The sense of well-being we feel after a massage is one reason some hospitals now offer it to patients as part of their treatment when preparing for surgery, or going through chemo, since it has been shown to help with anxiety, insomnia, and boosting immunity.

> **❝** *Caring for myself is not self-indulgent.*
> *Caring for myself is an act of survival."*
>
> - Audre Lorde

Besides its host of other benefits, massage involves allowing ourselves to be cared for in a comforting environment, and to establish a connection with our massage therapist. This connection is vital to us, and it is important for our physical, emotional, and mental well-being to be touched. I've had long rewarding relationships with my massage therapists, seeing the same one for years until they retired or moved. And a good massage therapist cares about you personally and works to earn your trust, learn your needs, and strives to restore your well-being.

Ask your doctor if massages are something you can add to your self-care routine, and ask for a recommendation. If your doctor doesn't work with someone, ask at your chiropractor, or at your yoga studio, or gym. Ask friends or your hair-stylist - they usually know a great massage therapist that they themselves rely on, and would be happy to recommend.

I once sent a friend to my massage therapist, and afterward she called me to report back. "I liked your massage therapist, but the place smelled like patchouli, and I hate patchouli."

It has to be the right fit, so you may want to visit the studio and have a quick consultation before scheduling your appointment. You want to learn whether the therapist works in a space where you will feel completely nurtured.

Getting a massage isn't a luxury; rather it's a necessity part of your health and wellness program for all of the reasons outlined above. Mostly though, massage is necessary because it's hard to live beautifully when you are in pain. Massage can help ease that pain and help you feel better about everything.

SIT STILL

I'm going to let you in on a little secret. For the longest time, I didn't like to meditate. I had been trying to do it for years, and the best I had managed was a "moving meditation" I learned at a weekend retreat many years ago. There, I'd walk a small labyrinth with my eyes almost closed, softly focused, able to see just enough that I didn't trip over something and cause myself bodily harm. As soon as the week was over, so was my meditating.

Years later, I began to do Trance Dance as my form of moving meditation. Blind-folded, with music playing, I could completely lose myself, be open to receiving insights, and enjoy freedom from my chattering mind. I did this for years, then I moved away from town and the long commute in traffic made it impractical for me to attend.

Now I am back to square one - sitting down and sitting still. I know meditation will be really good for me, but until now, I hadn't committed to it. I've even written a haiku about my attempts:

> How to meditate?
> Sitting seems a waste of time
> I could DO something!

What goes on in my head is utterly ridiculous. A pack of howler monkeys live there that only awakens when I get quiet. Things I didn't even know were a concern show up demanding attention the moment my butt hits the floor and I assume the position. After six months of twice-daily practice, 15-30 minutes each time, I have only just begun to have momentary glimpses of bliss, tiny 'gaps in between my thoughts,' and that feeling is so cool that I keep it up.

So why do I bother making myself sit to meditate? Well, I'll tell ya, first and foremost, I want to feel inner peace. More than anything, I really want to live the remainder of my life with equanimity. The benefits of simply sitting still are too good to ignore:

- ♥ Meditation reduces stress. Studies show an improved ability to regulate our emotions.
- ♥ It improves concentration. Meditation has been linked an increased ability to focus and remember.
- ♥ Meditation can encourage us to live a healthier lifestyle.
- ♥ Meditation increases our relaxation, which increases nitric oxide - remember that? It also helps improve our blood pressure and our immunity.
- ♥ It increases our happiness by increasing the brain activity responsible for positive emotions.
- ♥ The practice of meditation increases our self-awareness, and increases our acceptance of self and others.

I am the kind of woman who tries things just because they are good for me, and so I keep sitting. I've sat cross-legged on the sofa in the dark (liked it). I've sat outside on our balcony in a big wicker chair trying to ignore the sounds of traffic below me (did not like it). I've sat in bed, headboard supporting my back (liked it a lot).

Heaven knows, I even sat in the shower, warm water flowing over me as I waited for calm to come (once you figure out how not to drown yourself, it's great!). And I know calmness will come the more I practice. How do I know? I have faith.

To help you get inspired, let's 'bust some myths' about meditation:

1. Myth #1 - It's hard to do. With a little bit of instruction from a meditation teacher, it's easy and fun. It can be as simple as focusing on your breath, or repeating a mantra. Yes, that's where "OM" comes in. The challenge is we (I'm talking to myself here) often try too hard. Or get so distracted by our

thoughts that we think we are doing it wrong. Or we want immediate results.

2. Myth #2 - We must quiet our minds if we want to be successful. (As I wrote that sentence I saw the error in my thinking: it's not about being successful, this only creates more stress). When thoughts arise, as they will, see them as thoughts, don't judge them, and return to our breath or mantra.

    Dr. David Simon, from the Chopra Center, tells students, "The thought, I'm having thoughts, may be the most important thought you have ever thought. Before that, you probably thought you were your thoughts."

    The more often we practice, the more time we will spend in a state of awareness.

3. Myth # 3 - It takes years to become good at it. The Chopra Center states you can begin to experience benefits the first time you sit down to meditate. Science shows meditation affects the mind/body connection within weeks of beginning practice.

    In only eight weeks, studies have found growth in the parts of the brain dealing with empathy, memory, sense of self, and regulation of stress. Stress is a common feeling to those with ongoing illnesses, and eliminating it will be of great benefit to our whole body.

    Even "newbies" found that they slept well for the first time in years.

4. Assorted Myths -I thought meditation was a form of escapism, but I learned the goal isn't to tune-out the world, it is intended to tune-in to yourself, so you can be here now.

    People think they don't have time to meditate, but you only need a few minutes a day. Ignore social media for 15 minutes. Take a little time out of your lunch break. Skip the news and turn off the TV earlier. If all else fails, meditate sitting up in bed, lights dimmed, before going to sleep at night.

    I've had people ask if meditation was a religious ritual. No, it's just a mindfulness practice which will make you a happier person, no matter your religious affiliation, or lack of one.

THE HOW OF SITTING STILL

In an effort to learn more, I turned to The Chopra Center. The first thing I learned is some people do have more trouble sitting still and concentrating than others, and I was relieved to know I am not the only one.

Through practice, meditation will become easier. Just by noticing our thoughts, we expand our consciousness. It may feel like nothing happened, or you have spent the whole time trying not to think, but, hang in there, because meditation provides benefits even if we don't think we gain anything from that ten or fifteen minutes.

Some other things I do to help calm my over-active mind:

1. I've used both meditation music and nature sounds while learning to meditate. My favorite has turned out to be a 30-minute "mindfulness bell." It calls me back when my thoughts start wander too far.

2. Using coloring books. My sister and I used to buy each other intricate coloring books and relax together, coloring and having tea. Now, research shows coloring may be the best alternative to meditation. Many books are available now specifically for adults. I use it as an adjunct.

3. Spending time alone outdoors, sitting quietly and observing nature. There's no better place to zone out, and if you can take off your shoes and feel grass under your feet, all the better.

I am finally noticing results from my meditation. Inspired by this, I will keep at it. It's a worthy endeavor on many levels, and the health benefits are too good to ignore. Expanding our consciousness is something we can do for the rest of our lives, and an open mind is a sexy mind.

I hope you'll want to become one of the millions of people in the U.S. who meditate.

Consider Your Alternatives

We all have our cadre of doctors who dispense our prescriptions and track our symptoms and our progress, or lack thereof, but often with very little interdisciplinary awareness. I told my rheumatologist that my chiropractor had suggested I try a Paleo diet for a month, and I asked his opinion. He had none.

As I followed the diet, within weeks I noticed how GOOD I felt. I also noticed a lessening of the swelling and aching in my joints, and that I had more energy. I reported all of this to him on my next visit. While he agreed my hands and wrists did look much better, when I suggested enthusiastically, "You've got to tell your clients to try this!" he assured me that since it's all unsubstantiated, he couldn't.

Which brings me to my point: many healing modalities are available to us. I'm sure you've heard of most of these, but familiar practices are being applied in new ways. I have used every technique here, and all have helped me feel better.

*Disclaimer - None of these should be considered a replacement for conventional treatment of diseases, but they are a wonderful adjunct to our routine.

DIETITIANS AND NUTRITIONISTS

Let's start with the difference between the two: a Dietitian is a health professional who has university qualifications, which include a Master Degree in Nutrition and Dietetics. They are experts in prescribing therapeutic nutrition, and they are involved in the diagnoses and dietary treatment of many diseases such as food allergies, diabetes, and cancer.

Some states require Nutritionists to obtain an occupational license from a Board of Nutrition, while others allow individuals to practice without any previous education, training, or work experience.

However, there are also skilled Nutritionists who have completed University degrees in Food Science, Human Nutrition, or Food Technology. They normally work for food manufacturers, in research, or as food journalists. Since they don't generally have any professional practical training, they shouldn't be involved in the diagnosis or dietary treatment of diseases.

Know the qualifications of the one you see. Ask for referrals and recommendations from one of your doctors, or from a friend who also lives with chronic illness and is being successfully treated. Some things are too complex to figure out on your own, and it pays to seek out someone knowledgeable to help you.

Food is the building block of health and wellness, and probably our happiness. Many of our good memories are associated with food, and that's why people dislike the word diet, because it implies deprivation or restriction. Calling it an eating plan, or food guidelines, sounds much more neutral.

And, that's all it is, a suggested plan of foods to eat in order to feel our best. And, feeling great is the goal, right?

When the autoimmune disorder first flared up, and all of the comfort foods I prepared made me feel even worse, I realized that a food component was related to my symptoms. Nobody was talking about this very much then, and I found little information or online-support. I tried an Anti-Inflammatory Diet, which helped, but the joint pain and stiffness weren't abating.

Hoping an adjustment would help loosen things up, I went to see my chiropractor. When he couldn't find a way to offer relief, he suggested I try the Paleo Diet for a month and see what happened.

Just a few days earlier, a friend had bragged that he, his wife, and his brother, had all tried "this new Paleo Diet." I could tell the moment I saw him that he looked healthier. He also talked about how much fun it was, how good he felt, and how much he was enjoying doing the cooking!

The Universe was telling me something: following the guidelines I found online, I made some changes to my diet and in less than three weeks I felt good. Really good, for the first time in months! My hands weren't as swollen, and I could move my neck and shoulders with ease again.

A while later I stumbled upon the Primal Diet, a more flexible version of Paleo. I liked the fact it was a "lifestyle" of food and fitness. I enjoy the Primal fan-club and their participation - they post recipes with photos, and I've added a few favorite meals that are company worthy to my repertoire. I have been primarily primal for more than five years now, with only a few modifications and occasional cheats.

Some of us need very specific food plans, and you owe it to yourself and your loved ones to know them and follow them. For example, women with diabetes have guidelines they should learn and adhere to, because the results of long-term non-compliance for diabetics are frightening.

I just read statistics stating that up to 85% of amputations are preventable. This is where having a good dietitian on your team is going to be instrumental to your long-term well-being. Find someone qualified to help with your particular chronic illness and include them in your wellness-team.

> " *The natural healing force within each one of us is the greatest force in getting well. Our food should be our medicine. Our medicine should be our food."*
>
> - Hippocrates

REIKI THERAPY

The word 'reiki' is a set of Japanese characters that signify healing through the use of universal life force energy. Who among us with chronic illnesses wouldn't like more life force energy?

Reiki is a technique whereby a therapist synchronizes a client's energy field with a specific healthy, balanced vibration. Therapists may apply Reiki by either holding their hands slightly above the body or with a very light touch on the body. This activates natural healing and relaxation processes in our body, helping to restore us to balance and improved health.

I am lucky to have a friend who is a Reiki Master. I climb up on her table fully dressed, snuggle down, and get cozy, and before I know it an hour has passed. I usually fall asleep at some point, but always wake up right as she's finishing, more refreshed than after a whole night's sleep. We have a quick conversation and go over what she observed, and what I can do to support her work.

Carrie taught me that Bach Flower Essences work very well as a compliment to Reiki. They can provide overall support to the mind and body, and safely complement other therapeutic modalities. (Translation: they do not interfere with our medicines) They can be taken under the tongue, or in a glass of filtered water, in a hot bath, and even applied topically. I usually have a bottle of Rescue Remedy on hand at all times, just in case.

Unless you live in the middle-of-nowhere, you should be able to find a Reiki practitioner. Many massage therapists also study Reiki, so ask at your local massage or yoga studio if you haven't find one. If that doesn't work, try asking your hairstylist; they usually have a massage therapist they rely on and they may know a great Reiki practitioner or refer you to someone who does.

CHIROPRACTIC TREATMENT

I've always called my reliance on my chiropractor, my adjustment attitude. For more than thirty years, visiting a chiropractor has been one of my lifesavers. It helps restore my energy, my alignment, and my positive outlook on life.

Chiropractic care is based on the theory that proper alignment of our musculoskeletal structure, especially our spine, will help restore us to good health. I've used it for back pain, and that's probably what gets most of us in the door. I used it to keep me pain-free during the years I spent with my arms up, working with brushes and blow-dryers. My visits became indispensable when the connective-tissue disorder created stiffness in my neck and shoulders that hindered my work.

As I said earlier, it was my chiropractor who suggested I give the Paleo Diet a try to see if it would offer me relief. My trust in his instincts literally changed my life. We should all have health goals, we should know how we want to feel, and work toward it. This includes finding doctors to give us the tools to help our body function to its fullest potential.

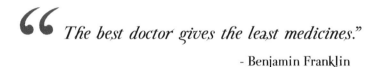

The best doctor gives the least medicines."

- Benjamin Franklin

Let's start with the benefits of chiropractic care: It's a drug-free way to help clients reach their health goals. You may know it best as a treatment for back pain. While it is used primarily as pain relief for our muscles, joints, bones, and connective tissue, it's also good for headaches, ear aches, arthritis, asthma, blood pressure, osteoarthritis, fibromyalgia, organ function, and surgery prevention.

Chiropractors realize that neck pain doesn't just affect your neck; left untreated it can spill over and affect your whole life. I've long since learned that an appointment offers immediate relief, and emotional support. Rather than wait to see if things will improve, I call and get an adjustment for both my body and my spirit.

Chiropractic care is used in conjunction with conventional medicine more frequently now. Hospitals have chiropractors on staff. Most health insurance now covers visits to the chiropractor to help keep us well, and to avoid costlier, more extensive treatment down the road.

I just visited my friend Chuck Karam, DC, to try a new technique called "active release" used to break up soft tissue distortion in the fascia. He said there are many techniques, more than a hundred, and he looks at what is right for each patient.

After observing me and how I moved, he worked on my neck and shoulder, my hips, and even on the joints in my hands, which had been hurting for more than a month. Nobody has ever worked on my hands, and it made a huge difference. A week later, my hands still feel better. This technique can offer much relief to those of us with connective-tissue disorders.

> " *Keeping your body healthy is an expression of gratitude to the whole cosmos - the trees, the clouds, everything"*
>
> - Thich Nhat Hanh

ACUPUNCTURE

I must confess I haven't been to the acupuncturist for a few years, and now that I'm thinking about it, I am going to remedy my hiatus. I used to go because I was bothered by allergies that caused congestion headaches and created a sinus infection every winter. All of that is now a thing of the past.

Whenever I talk about visiting an acupuncturist, people usually respond with, "Oh, I hate needles!" Well, there are needles, and then there are needles. The ones used in this acupuncture are the furthest thing from what is used to give us an injection or to draw blood. Apples and oranges, seriously.

I enjoyed many things about a visit to the clinic, but the one I savored the most was the novelty of everything. An exotic quality intrigues and relaxes me the moment I walk in the door. And it never gets old. All of this is so different than our normally streamlined, sterile doctor's offices.

Acupuncture is often used as an adjunct to other forms of treatment, such as relieving nausea and vomiting caused by chemotherapy. It is also used for fibromyalgia, osteoarthritis, and headaches, including migraines. In Traditional Chinese Medicine, it is believed energy meridians run through our bodies, and the needles are inserted at places that would specifically stimulate corresponding body parts.

Thus, treatment for allergies could be needles inserted into the backs of your hands or top of your feet, as well as between your eyebrows and beside your nose. After treatment you may feel either relaxed or energetic, since everyone reacts differently. And you can even feel different from one visit to the next. If your symptoms don't improve after a couple weeks, consider it may not be the right treatment for you.

Licensed acupuncturists are required to use sterile, single-use, disposable needles in order to keep you safe from disease. You should ask if they follow this practice during your consultation. And, most states require certification by the Commission for Acupuncture and Oriental Medicine.

Ask your doctor first if this treatment would be all right for you. Then ask people you know for a recommendation, or look for an acupuncture academy and make an appointment for an initial consultation.

My visits to the acupuncture clinic have been more like spa treatments than medical treatments. If you decide to give it a try, I hope you benefit greatly from it.

My experiences with all of these "alternative" modalities throughout the years have been wonderful, leaving me feeling well, and very well cared for. There's always more we can do to feel our best, and these all felt like a reward, a gift to myself.

SICK AND TIRED... & TRAVELING

We arrived home from our vacation with friends on our motorcycles last night after driving for almost 15 hours. We finally crawled into bed at midnight, and I made myself crawl back out of bed at 7:00 a.m. I would probably have stayed in bed all day, but I had things that needed to be done.

Was our vacation wonderful? Yes. And no.

It was harder than I ever let on. For the last few years, each time we take one of our group trips, there comes a point toward the end of the trip where I think, "I can't do this again, it's too much."

This time that thought came early and kept coming back. And this time, it was followed by, "I just can't keep up with them anymore."

The realization made me overwhelmingly sad for a day or two, but I will find another way to travel that is more suited to my health. I'm sure you've had the same feeling; it's challenging to accept we aren't in control of everything, no matter how much we try.

On this trip, as much as I paid attention to my needs, I still got off my (necessarily rigid) schedule. Medicines didn't get taken on time. I'd get caught up in the party atmosphere and have one more cocktail than I should. I'd try a bite of this, and a little bit of that, and I ended up not feeling well.

For the first time ever, I was so ill that I held the whole group up - I had to keep stopping to run to a bathroom: in a dirty gas station, in a seedy bar, in a convenience store, a restaurant, and finally in a nice clean Starbucks. I could write a book about bathrooms across the country, but I'd rather not.

The good news: our friends all understand that shit happens.
The bad news: I was sick, and I felt ridiculous.

Since I'd never been sick on a trip before, it took me by surprise. And there was nothing I could do except let it run its course.

Sometimes all we can do is go with the flow. I do not want to give up traveling by motorcycle. It's what we do with our group of friends, and what we love to do most as a couple. However, I will find a way that will serve me better. I don't know what that will be yet, but I am open to it.

> 66 *The secret of health for both mind and body*
> *is not to mourn for the past, worry about the*
> *future, or anticipate troubles, but to live in*
> *the present moment wisely and earnestly."*
>
> - Buddha

How can I, how can we all, take the best care of ourselves when we travel, so that each trip is a fun-filled exploration and adventure? By following the Boy Scout motto: Be Prepared.

Being prepared means knowing how your body responds at its worst and having what you need, in case that happens. We should do our best to avoid getting to our worst-case scenarios, but if that doesn't work, then all we can do is accept it and take care of ourselves.

Plan ahead: Have all of your medicines with you. Actually, have more than you will need. What if you were delayed a day or two, or even more? Be sure your prescriptions have a refill remaining, in case you needed to have them transferred. If you don't already have a pill-case for traveling, get one. They are lifesavers. I finally admitted I needed it, and bought one organized for morning/mid-day/evening. Now I can always tell what I've taken, and what I haven't. No more missed doses because things are off schedule!

An ounce of prevention: I carry Tums, Pepcid, Immodium, Papaya digestive enzymes, and Ibuprofen. They work for me, and there's no search for a drug-store in an unfamiliar city. What do you need to have on hand? I also bring a paperback book even if I don't expect to have time to read it. It beats sitting in a hotel bathroom staring at the wallpaper or baseboards.

Damage control: This is where muscle-relaxers, anti-anxiety medications, and the like come in for me. For you it may be painkillers, migraine medicines, or all-of-the above. What do you need to have with you in case all else has failed?

If that happens, try to remember that it's really not the worst thing that could happen. Inconvenient? Sure. A waste of time? It would seem that way. But you are still here on the planet, and you are still on vacation.

Reality check: Because of this recent vacation, I realized some types of trips may be better than others for certain types of chronic illnesses. A vacation with multiple-destinations and a tight schedule is no longer the ideal one for me. Being able to take things at my body's pace would be better suited to "how I roll" these days.

Own it: I've talked about co-dependence elsewhere, but it bears repeating. If I need to stay in the room all day, I encourage my sweetheart to have fun and come back and tell me all about it later. Feeling bad doesn't mean we need to make others stay with us (unless we are severely ill and need help). Just because I am missing out (and with a good book, I never feel that way) doesn't mean my partner needs to. And, since I love him, I wouldn't ask him to.

Bottom line: Even people without chronic illnesses become ill while on vacation. They catch bugs on airplanes, they contract tourista south of the border, altitude sickness in the mountains, even allergic reactions to air pollution in Paradise.

Remember, these things are all part of being human. Be gentle with yourself. Be prepared. And go have fun!

YOU, UNLIMITED

❝ *The garden of the world has no limits, except in your mind."*

- Rumi

When living with chronic illnesses, it's important to stay open-minded and remember that change is the only constant. That's good news because it means that things can always get better.

When our thoughts about things change, we will change. That is, of course, unless we prefer the comfort and the excuse that our illnesses afford us.

Right about now, I imagine you've stopped and thought, "Hey, wait a minute! What do you mean by that?"

Let me put it this way. There have certainly been times I didn't want to do something, and used an illness as my excuse. Our illnesses can allow us to avoid commitments, obligations, and other things we really don't want to do, or things we are afraid to try. Illness provides a legitimate excuse to give both ourselves and others; an excuse that we won't be judged on, or blamed for, at least not for a while.

Being chronically ill can be:

- ♥ A way to get sympathy and attention.
- ♥ Used to manipulate and control others, or to be a martyr.
- ♥ Used as an excuse to get out of doing things we don't want to do.
- ♥ An excuse not to try new things or to give up on our dreams.

If you happen to find yourself using your illness as an excuse, ask yourself these questions:

- ♥ WHEN do you use it to get out of doing things?
- ♥ What is the REAL reason you don't want to do this thing?
- ♥ What is it you are AVOIDING?
- ♥ Why don't you feel you can tell the TRUTH?

Love Note: Use this as an opportunity to learn more about yourself, not to beat yourself up. Every bit of this is judgment-free, and an opportunity to love yourself a little bit more.

I am calling attention to this because I did it, too. One day I realized what I was doing, and I've got to say, it was a startling awareness. I didn't want to be the kind of woman to make excuses, or not tell the truth, especially to myself. And I didn't want to avoid doing things.

Here's the good news: when you look at the things in your life you use illness to avoid, you've faced something really important. And you will have gained freedom, energy, self-love, and confidence.

What if, in facing your "why," you establish strong boundaries that will allow you to take better care of yourself?

What if, in telling the truth, you reveal more of who you really are and your relationships grow stronger?
What if, in choosing to be honest, you find out what you really want in your life?

What if healing this schism could begin, or accelerate, your own healing process?

This is your life and unless you plan to sit on the sidelines and live it vicariously, you must learn to live exactly the way you want. And, what better time to learn than right now?

When I told myself the truth, my life got simpler. I got clear on what I did and didn't want. I decided what I would make time for, and what I wouldn't anymore. I'm learning to ask for exactly what I want or need. I practice making all of my decisions to take care of my health and well-being, first.

It was an eye-opener to realize that if I continually chose not to do things because I didn't think I could, or because I was feeling too tired, I would never do anything. We must not allow illness to limit us. It is amazing what we can accomplish by taking small, even tiny, steps.

By doing just that, I've built an inventory of reference points to remind myself I can do something even when I think I can't. As I've done more things I didn't think I could, my capabilities have grown and so has my confidence. Despite living with multiple chronic illnesses, I enjoy my life.

(To be clear: I do not have a debilitating illness - that's another story entirely, my heartfelt compassion to you if you are one of the women who do. I am talking only about my experience with the constant state of tiredness, achiness, and lack of zeal that accompanies many chronic illnesses.)

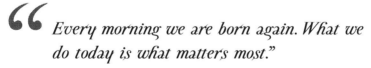

Every morning we are born again. What we do today is what matters most."

- Buddha

Chronic illnesses may often present us with limitations, but it's important to know the difference between limitations and the limiting beliefs we set for ourselves. Or allow others set for us unconsciously. The trick is not to let your "limits" limit you, but to learn to use them as a springboard.

Because of my dietary restrictions, I've become a much more creative cook. I love being in the kitchen trying new recipes, and by doing so, I keep myself feeling well and not deprived in the least! I miss going out to socialize the way I used to, but that's led to smaller, more intimate get-togethers, and deepening friendships.

Living with chronic illnesses also inspired me to pursue my dreams. Where will it lead you?

❝ *On the long journey of human life, faith is the best of companions."*

- Buddha

I once heard a line in a movie that really resonated for me, "For such a spiritual person, you have very little faith." That was me, but everything I did in my quest to feel better has ultimately led me to a place where I have faith. Faith in both myself and in a power greater than myself.

My connection to a higher power was always somewhere between non-existent and amorphous, at best. As I began to institute all of my daily practices, I grew to realize something Deepak Chopra said in a private talk I attended, "God is a Responsive Universe."

I had wishes and intentions. I took care of myself as a demonstration of my intentions and took actions toward my goals, being grateful all along the way, and I am now living the life I envisioned. You need to have faith in whoever or whatever that power is for you.

And you need to maintain an attitude of gratitude, no matter what. We gain strength by being grateful for what we have, and by focusing on all we are grateful for. Remember, everything is always changing, which means it can always get better, and we can always feel better. Perhaps we can heal completely. Our happiness depends on our thoughts, and what we choose to focus on.

In my experience, as I made slow, steady changes, I saw things in a different way. And as I saw things differently, each change led me to the next one. Before I knew it, I could look back and see how far I had come.

I wish the same thing for you. I hope these pages have provided some ideas and thoughts to inspire you. You'll surprise yourself with what you are capable of doing. You'll be astonished at how quickly a few small changes add up to big results. You can indeed live a beautiful, sexy life, even while living with chronic illness!

> *If you realized how beautiful you are, you would fall at your own feet."*
>
> - Byron Katie

A beautiful Buddhist meditation

Just sit. Notice where you feel hard, and sit with that.

In the middle of that hardness, you'll find anger; sit with that.

Go to the center of the anger and you'll probably come to sadness.

Stay with the sadness until it turns to vulnerability.

Keep sitting with what comes up; the deeper you dig, the more tender you become.

Raw fear can open into the wide expanse of genuineness, compassion, gratitude, and acceptance in the present moment.

A tender heart appears naturally when you are able to stay present.

From your heart, you can see the true pigment of the sky.

You can see the vibrant yellow of the sunflower and the deep blue of your daughter's eyes.

A tender heart doesn't block out rainclouds, or tears, or dying sunflowers.

Allow both beauty and sadness to touch you. This is love, not fear.

Acknowledgements

To the unsinkable Lee Moczygemba, a heartfelt thanks for the important part you play in my life.

My loving gratitude to my family - Lynn, Andee, Elizabeth, my son Jason who shares my passion for the arts, Delaine, Daddy-O and Ginny, and Laurie W

My tribe - Holly (you too, Mike), Denise, Carole, Leisa, Gina, Candy, Sheri, Jillian (you too, Rob).

My doctors - Laurence Tokaz, MD, and my wonderful NP, Pam Garza, Beth Miller, MD, and Gwendolyn Miller, MD, Gary Seghi, DC, and Eduardo Cepeda, MD.

For contributing your knowledge - Holly Nastasi, M.Ed., Chuck Karam, DC, and Carrie Laymon.

All of my dear clients who have listened and encouraged, especially Laurie M, Bobbi S, Susan T, Karen M, and Susan L.

Those who have inspired - Philip S, Jason A, Bill and Linda, Ron M, Zan, Ted and Jason, Steven, and the Bella Salon family.

To Ilene and BlogathonATX for showing me where to start.

To Linda S and her wonderful YBBBP for giving me a plan.

To Jihan and my Quantum Shift Quest family-of-the-heart for providing the structure I needed.

To Cynthia Stone at TREATY OAK PUBLISHERS, and to Aralyn Hughes for introducing us.

Special thanks to Julia Cameron, Seth Godin, Tara Mohr, Leanne Shirtliffe, Debbie Rosas, Gretchen Rubin, and Mark Sisson for their quotes.

Resources

Books that inspired, in no particular order:

Sick and Tired of Feeling Sick and Tired, Paul J. Donohue Ph.D. and Mary E. Seigel Ph.D., W.W. Norton & Co, 2000

Life Disrupted, Laurie Edwards, Walker and Company, NY 2008

In the Kingdom of the Sick, Laurie Edwards, Bloomsbury, 2013

Brain on Fire: My Month of Madness, Susannah Calahan, Simon & Schuster, 2012

Crazy Sexy Cancer Tips, Sheryl Crow & Kris Carr, Guilford, CT, 2007

A Return to Love, Marianne Williamson, Harper Collins, 1992

The Art of Happiness, The Dalai Lama & Howard C. Cutler M.D., Riverhead Books, 1998

the life changing magic of tidying up, marie kondo, Ten Speed Press,2014

The Complete Works, Florence Scovel Shinn, Dover Publications, 2010

The Artist's Way, Julia Cameron, Jeremy P. Tarcher/Perigee Books, 1992

Playing Big, Tara Mohr, Gotham Books, 2014

The Desire Map, Danielle LaPorte, Sounds True, Inc. 2014

The Power of Habit, Charles Duhigg, Random House, 2012

Eat, Pray, Love, Elizabeth Gilbert, Penguin Books, 2006

Big Magic, Elizabeth Gilbert, Riverhead Books, 2013

The Happiness Project, Gretchen Rubin, Harper Paperbacks, 2011

Awaken the Giant Within, Tony Robbins, Fireside/Simon & Schuster, 1991

Bird by Bird, Anne Lamott, Pantheon Books, 1994

Food and Healing, Anne Marie Colbin, A Ballentine Book, 1986

The Omnivore's Dilemma, Michael Pollan, Penguin Press, 2006

Tribes: We Need You to Lead Us, Seth Godin, Penguin Group, 2008

The Art of Stillness, Pico Ayer, TED Books Simon & Schuster, 2014

Online content that always inspires me (again, in no particular order):

Marieforleo.com

BookMama.com and Linda Sivertsen

jkrowling.com

apartmenttherapy.com

gretchenrubin.com

Juliacameronlive.com

daniellelaporte.com especially her #Truthbombs

marksdailyapple.com and Mark Sisson

Zenhabits.com

Ironicmom.com by Leanne Shirtliffe

Michaelpollan.com His movies, and books.

Webmd.com

TED.com, TED talks on YouTube

https://Nianow.com, Debbie Rosas - Moving our body in meaningful ways.

Sethgodin.com

drweil.com and Dr. Andrew Weil

Terrywahls.com and her Wahls Protocol for MS

Barry Schwartz talks on TED.com

sufferingthesilence.com An online chronic illness community.

Excellent reads:

In the Kingdom of the Sick by Laurie Edwards

Life Disrupted by Laurie Edwards

Crazy, Sexy, Cancer by Kris Carr

You Don't Look Sick by Joy Selak and Steven Oberman

Sick and Tired of Feeling Sick and Tired by Paul Donoghue and Mary E. Siegel

Dying to Be Me: My Journey from Cancer, to Near Death, to True Healing by Anita Moorjani

How to Live Well with Chronic Pain and Illness by Toni Bernhard

How to Be Sick: A Buddhist Guide for the Chronically Ill by Toni Bernhard

Tales from the Bed: On Living, Dying, and Having it All by Jenifer Estes

KNOWING: a spiritual memoir of healing and hope by Ginger Blair

Money: A Love Story by Kate Northrup (helped me get a handle on my anxiety over all of those pesky medical bills)

About the Author

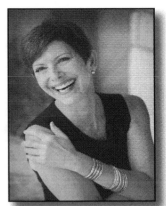

Donna O'Klock grew up in Bayport, Long Island, NY, the oldest of five girls. With fond memories of visiting Texas by train as a child, she moved to Austin with her son in 1978. After a brief stint working at the Austin Public Library, she opened her first hairstyling salon in 1980, right next door to Grok Books.

In addition to her salon clientele, she has done hair and makeup for independent films, television, theater, political campaigns, and local photographers. She is now retired from the beauty industry.

Donna is also a blogger, posting at SexyPast60.com and DamnedGypsy.com, and on 1010ParkPlace, an online magazine celebrating women over 45. She lives with her fiancé, and, along with their shared passion for travel and motorcycles, she is an avid photographer and cook, currently striving to perfect the art of gluten-free pastries.

Author photo by Korey Howell

Made in the USA
San Bernardino, CA
29 October 2018